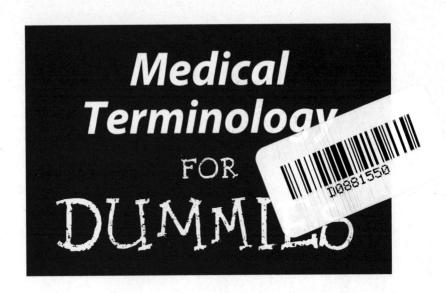

Medical
Terminology
FOR
DUMMIES

by Beverley Henderson, CMT and Jennifer Dorsey

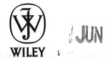

WILEY

Wiley Publishing, Inc.

Medical Terminology For Dummies®

Published by
Wiley Publishing, Inc.
111 River St.
Hoboken, NJ 07030-5774
www.wiley.com

Copyright © 2009 by Wiley Publishing, Inc., Indianapolis, Indiana

Published by Wiley Publishing, Inc., Indianapolis, Indiana

Published simultaneously in Canada

For general information on our other products and services, please contact our Customer Care Department within the U.S. at 877-762-2974, outside the U.S. at 317-572-3993, or fax 317-572-4002.

For technical support, please visit www.wiley.com/techsupport.

Wiley also publishes its books in a variety of electronic formats. Some content that appears in print may not be available in electronic books.

Library of Congress Control Number: 2008939701

ISBN: 978-0-470-27965-6

Manufactured in the United States of America

10 9 8 7 6 5 4 3

WILEY

About the Authors

Beverley Henderson, CMT has enjoyed a lifelong career in the medical field. Working in Ontario hospitals for 45 years, she also has more than 40 years' experience in medical terminology and transcription. She has managed the medical transcription unit of a large acute-care hospital and has taught medical terminology to adult learners at the university level. Beverley is a Certified Medical Transcriptionist with the American Association for Medical Transcription. She was Director of Health Sciences Faculty and MT Course Coordinator at an online medical terminology and transcription school, where she developed course curricula and helped write and produce a series of medical terminology teaching videos. Now an empty-nester, she lives in Hamilton with her husband of 35 years.

Jennifer Dorsey has been a writer and editor for 11 years. She has worked for publishers both large and small, mainly focusing her efforts on development editing and acquisitions. In 2005 she turned her focus to writing and has worked on several projects, including revisions of four popular how-to titles from Entrepreneur Press, most notably How to Start Your Own Medical Claims Billing Business. She has also written magazine articles for Indiana Business Magazine, Indianapolis Monthly, and California Homes. In 1997 she received her B.A. in journalism from Saint Mary-of-the-Woods College, the oldest Catholic liberal arts college for women in the United States. She is currently pursuing her M.A. in English and is a member of the adjunct faculty at Saint Louis University. She lives in Illinois with her husband and son.

Dedication

Beverley Henderson: This book is dedicated to my friends and family. To the co-workers who have become my friends, gathered over a 40-year span while working at the Henderson Hospital, Joseph Brant Memorial Hospital, and recently St. Joseph's Hospital and Hamilton Health Sciences. Special thanks to close friends Pat Harmer and Isabelle Holland for their ongoing support, entertaining lunches, and hilarious stories.

To my parents, Mary and Bill Hunter, I'm only sorry they are not here to read this book. To my father, who taught me to challenge my brain on a daily basis. To my mother, whose high expectations of me kept my feet firmly on the ground. To my daughter Michele, who showed me that it's never too late to change careers. To my son Ian, who is living proof that brains, good looks, courtesy, and respect do exist in just one man.

To my husband Richard, my Scottish "diamond in the rough," the love of my life. His steadfast love, understanding, and above all, patience, has allowed me always and without question, to follow my career dreams down any road I ever wanted.

Jennifer Dorsey: For the Diva, who is set to make her debut the same week as this book. Who knew that so much joy could happen all at once. Mommy loves you.

Acknowledgments

Beverley Henderson: My sincere thanks to Lindsay Lefever for having the faith and trust in my medical knowledge to take me on the Wiley bandwagon as the old "new kid on the block." Never in my wildest dreams did I imagine myself accomplishing a feat of this magnitude. I thank Lindsay for giving me the opportunity to write about a subject that has been a large part of my career for many years. I am truly honored to be included in the accomplishments of Wiley publications.

To my "partner in crime" in this endeavor, Jen Dorsey. I could not have done this without her. With her past experiences in writing, Jen has coached me through this new experience. Her patience and understanding, not to mention her answers to my never-ending questions, went above and beyond the call of duty. I hope to have the opportunity of working with Jennifer again in the future.

Jennifer Dorsey: Writing this book has been a dream come true for me. After working with some wonderful people as an acquisitions editor for Wiley (many moons ago), I was so thrilled to be asked back as a writer. I hope this is the beginning of another beautiful friendship.

Speaking of beautiful friendships, thanks to my co-author Beverly Henderson. Her medical knowledge is the heart of this book, and her passion really shows.

Big thanks go out to my talented acquisitions editor, Lindsay Lefever, for having faith that we could pull this off. She's an editorial guardian angel. Lindsay, I'm ready to start on the next book whenever you are. Corbin Collins, our fabulous project editor, has shown us patience and graciousness beyond measure. And he's still talking to us, which is pretty great considering he's a cool guy who likes Tom Waits! Innumerable thanks go out to all of the editorial and production folks, graphic artists, proofreaders, and indexers who make us look pretty darn good. You guys rock! Props also go to some old friends at Wiley, Megan Saur and Barry Pruett, who were kind enough to let me come play for a while before I headed to parts west. I'll always be grateful for the opportunities.

To my friends at home and on both coasts, my thanks for all of the email encouragement that got me through many a long night. Special thanks go out to my martini-loving ladies from the OC — Michelle, Rebekah, Erin, and Vicky. I miss you all every day! Also, special thanks to my Woodsie friends who make Mother Theodore Guerin proud every day by being very successful at what they do, socially aware when it counts, and just plain fabulous women.

My family is my support system without which I could not have survived the last few months. Thanks to all of my wonderful babysitters — Grandmas Rosie and Mickie, Beth, and Aunt Sandy in particular — who saved me on more than one occasion. Thanks to my awesome, funny, delightfully precocious son Will who has more brains and charm than James Bond (and knows it). He keeps me laughing and reminds me of what is most precious in life. Most importantly, thank you so much to my wonderful husband, Mike, who loves me no matter what crazy project I get us involved in ("Hey! Let's do a little kitchen renovation while I write the book!") and who has always believed this is the right path from the start.

Publisher's Acknowledgments

We're proud of this book; please send us your comments through our Dummies online registration form located at www.dummies.com/register/.

Some of the people who helped bring this book to market include the following:

Acquisitions, Editorial, and Media Development

Project Editor: Corbin Collins

Acquisitions Editor: Lindsay Lefevere

Copy Editor: Corbin Collins

Assistant Editor: Erin Calligan Mooney

Technical Editor: Gallaudet Howard

Senior Editorial Manager: Jennifer Ehrlich

Editorial Supervisor and Reprint Editor: Carmen Krikorian

Art Coordinator: Alicia B. South

Editorial Assistants: Joe Niesen, Jennette ElNaggar, David Lutton

Cartoons: Rich Tennant
(www.the5thwave.com)

Composition Services

Project Coordinator: Kristie Rees

Layout and Graphics: Melissa K. Jester, Sarah E. Philippart, Christine Williams

Special Art: Kathryn Born, LifeARTS

Proofreader: Sossity R. Smith

Indexer: Cheryl Duksta

Publishing and Editorial for Consumer Dummies

Diane Graves Steele, Vice President and Publisher, Consumer Dummies

Joyce Pepple, Acquisitions Director, Consumer Dummies

Kristin Ferguson-Wagstaffe, Product Development Director, Consumer Dummies

Ensley Eikenburg, Associate Publisher, Travel

Kelly Regan, Editorial Director, Travel

Publishing for Technology Dummies

Andy Cummings, Vice President and Publisher, Dummies Technology/General User

Composition Services

Gerry Fahey, Vice President of Production Services

Debbie Stailey, Director of Composition Services

Contents at a Glance

Table of Contents

Part IV: Let's Get Some Physiology Terminology 187

Introduction

● ●

Welcome to *Medical Terminology For Dummies!* Consider this your personal, private course in the study of the medical terms used everyday in doctor's offices, hospitals, clinics, billing and insurance companies, labs, and even pharmacies. This is a personal grand tour through not only the world of medical terminology, but also through your own body.

You'll find as you read this book that learning medical terms is a two-part proposition. First, you've got to master the landscape of language itself. Don't worry, though — there will be no quiz. We just want you to better understand how to both create and break down words. Once you get to know more about prefixes, suffixes, and root words, you can do darn near anything with the terminology. For example, you can go inside the body to discover the terms that match up with different systems, diseases, procedures, and pharmaceutical products.

Mastering medical terminology involves more than just memorizing. Exploring these terms and how they can be created will unlock not only medical mysteries for you, but great opportunities as well.

About This Book

Getting to know the world of medical terminology can get a bit repetitive at times. That's why we decided to break the book down into several parts about all kinds of different things. You start by getting the back story of terminology — the history and the players involved with bringing this "language" to the masses. Then you get into the nitty-gritty of how words are formed and all about word parts, usage, pronunciation, and recognition. Finally, you take a gander at all the different body systems and the words associated with them. We even threw in some bonus top ten lists at the end that we hope you find useful.

There's a lot to learn about medical terminology, we admit, but we'll be right there with you for the whole wild, crazy ride.

Keep in mind that this is not a giant textbook of terms, nor is it a dictionary. Those are both great resources, and we recommend you pick up both if you are a medical professional. This is a friendly take on the topic, and our main goal is to show you the basics of how these words are made so that you can go out in the big, bad world and master the creation and use of medical terms on your own terms. We're not giving you a fish, we're teaching you to fish.

Conventions Used in This Book

Truly, the best way to make sense of terminology (because it *is* like a language of its own in many respects) is to approach it as you would a foreign language. But we want you to feel comfortable with the concept of how a term is formed before you get crazy with your flashcards and recall devices. That's why you see many chapters about language and medical terminology's place in it.

You will notice we also make extensive use of lists in this book. We do this for your sanity. Be honest: Wouldn't you rather be able to study these terms in organized, easy-to-find lists and tables rather than picking through long, boring paragraphs trying to find the words you need to learn? We thought so.

Once you get the hang of medical terms and how they are formed, we change gears a little bit and jump right into the systems of the body. Each system chapter tells you a bit about how that particular body system works, to give you some context for its words. We aren't doctors, so we try our best to explain things using simple language. That means you might see words like *pee* and *poo* from time to time. We figure you're knee-deep in official-sounding terms here, so it doesn't hurt to lighten up once in a while.

As we said, there are a lot of lists. But in the text, we try and put new terms in italics where we define them, to make them easier to spot.

Don't be alarmed by those little pictures you see peppering the pages of this book. Feel free to be distracted, however — that's the point. We want you to stop and look at these great kernels of knowledge as you go through the book.

Marks concrete tips and tricks that you can put to use in giving you more control over your medical life.

Highlights passages that are good to keep in mind when mastering medical terminology.

Alerts you to common mistakes that can trip you up in your medical terminology studies.

This icon indicates you are about to read an interesting tidbit about the Greek heritage behind the terms you are learning.

Ditto here. This icon points you back to the Latin roots that helped make these terms possible.

This icon indicates something cool and perhaps a little offbeat from the discussion at hand.

Foolish Assumptions

We are assuming you fall into one of these categories:

- ✔ A medical student hoping to get a jumpstart on general terminology before that first big quiz.
- ✔ A medical professional looking to brush up on terms if you're a bit out of practice or just want to know more about how these terms are made.
- ✔ A curious adult interested in speaking your doctor's language and learning more about the terms that describe how your body functions.

No matter what possessed you to pick up this book, we hope it gives you the terminology boost you need for your particular circumstances. The human body has hundreds and hundreds of working parts, and they all have names. Moreover, there are names for all kinds of associated terms relating to functions, conditions, diseases, pathology, and even pharmacology. It's a whole lot, we grant you. But you are eager, right? And no amount of 50-cent words frighten you away from your goal: to become a medical terminology Zen master. You can do it, Grasshopper.

How This Book Is Organized

We don't mess around with much extraneous here in *For Dummies* land. You want to know the most important info in a friendly, easy-to-read manner, and we want to give it to you. Everybody wins.

This book starts at the most logical beginning, the background of medical terminology, and gets into where it all came from, who had a hand in developing it, and how it morphed into the modern version we use today. Then, you revisit grammar school briefly and read about word parts, their meanings, and how they all work together to make a cohesive word. If you hated grammar in school, don't fear. It isn't painful, and we think you'll find it interesting to read the story behind the terms. We promise: Words you may have taken for granted will reveal themselves in a whole new light, and, as a result, your "aha!" light bulb will be going off a lot.

Once that happens, the book takes you right into the human body for a grand tour of systems and the terms that go with them. Finally, you'll wind down with some useful top ten lists of great resources, word-building activities, and recall devices. By the time you turn that last page, we know you'll feel confident and ready to talk root words and eponyms with the best of them.

Part I: Living for Linguistics

To start your journey, you'll jump into the history of medical terminology and find out a bit about how the whole big, crazy mess evolved into something people use everyday in doctor's offices, hospitals, clinics, insurance and billing companies, and even pharmacies.

Believe it or not, medical terms didn't just magically appear on tablets dropped from the sky. Someone put a great deal of thought into how they would be created. You'll find out all about the Greeks, the Romans, and even more modern medical gurus for whom many terms are named.

Once you get a little history under your belt, you will get familiar with the basic three building blocks of words: roots, prefixes, and suffixes. You can mix and match these like a shell game and get a different word every time. You'll wrap up your terminology basic training by taking a look at pronunciation, usage, plurals, and multiples.

Part II: Mapping Words and Bodies

Here's where you start to fine-tune your terminology skills. This part takes you through the vast world of prefixes, suffixes, and how words are formed. Before you know it, you'll be amazing your friends with all your word-building party tricks. And, just like mapping a word, you can start to think more about how those terms relate to the universe that is your body. You hit some quick highlights of your body's systems and functions, learning how they work together, before moving on to some more detailed explanations of the terms associated with those systems.

Part III: In Terms of Anatomy

This is where the fun starts, the big daddy chapters in which you find out all about different body systems and the words that help describe them. From your infrastructure (also known around some parts as your skeletal system) to your muscles, senses, and *integumentary* (a fancy word for hair, skin, and nails) system, you'll find hundreds of words and word parts used to describe them. Here you read about many of them in terms of basic description, pathology, testing and procedures, and pharmacology.

Part IV: Let's Get Some Physiology Terminology

Keeping up with the internal dynamics of medical terms, you move on to body systems that are a bit more physiological. The heart — literally — of the operation is your cardiovascular system. It's helped out by your respiratory system, which helps you breathe and provides oxygen to the blood. The gastrointestinal system is full of words describing how what you eat becomes what you expel. All your hormones and crazy chemicals are kept in check by your endocrine system, while your nervous system also pitches in to manage body chemicals and reactions. Your body is like a giant circus, and the terms used to describe it are the fliers you follow to make sense of it all.

Part V: Name That Plumbing

Call us crazy, but we think your pee and babymaking parts are important enough for a whole part in this book. Hey, why not dedicate some major space to the systems that purge your body of toxins and provide the key to maintaining the world population? Reading this part, you get to know everything you always wanted to about your urinary tract and then — hang on to your hat — you get a refresher course in Sex Ed. Of course, there are tons of terms to help you along the way and, like the other systems, they describe body parts, conditions, diseases, procedures, and drugs.

Part VI: The Part of Tens

Just to make sure you've covered all the bases, be sure to check out this part that is chock-full of fun tidbits. We cover where to look for great resources, fun word-building activities, and some commonly used mnemonic devices.

Where to Go from Here

By all means, if you're feeling spunky you can jump right into this book at any point and start working on your terminology savvy. Mastering the how and why of medical terms is sometimes as important as learning the terms themselves, which is why we put those chapters first. But by all means, feel free to hunt and peck the sections that are most useful to you.

Be bold. Be brave. And, most importantly, proceed through this book with confidence. Once you get the hang of how these words are made, you'll have no problem committing them to memory and to your daily life.

Part I
Living for Linguistics

The 5th Wave
By Rich Tennant

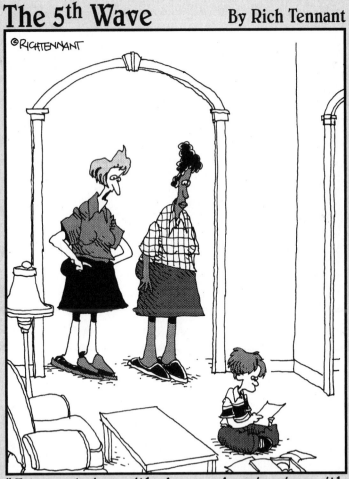

"I know being with dogs and swimming with dolphins have proven therapeutic for ASDs, but when my doctor suggested Hippotherapy for our son I said there's no way he's getting in a mud hole with a giant pig."

In this part . . .

Lay some groundwork for medical terminology before you get involved with individual body systems. Chapter 1 gives you an overview of the basic building blocks of learning terminology. Chapter 2 provides you with a background dossier on terminology and its history, whereas Chapter 3 familiarizes you with the all-important concept of the root word. Chapter 4 takes you through the world of multiples and plurals, and Chapter 5 introduces you to tips and tricks for pronunciation and usage.

Chapter 1

Scrubbing In to Master
Medical Terminology

Did you realize that when you picked up this book, you were beginning a journey into a whole new language? Don't worry — you haven't grabbed *Greek For Dummies* by mistake — it's all English, or at least "English." But once you get deep into the world of medical terms, you will find that it is a whole new way of speaking. Your journey will indeed take you to ancient Greece as well as to Rome. You will meet some of the pioneers of the medical world. You will gain entrance into a whole new world: your body. All of those confusing terms you hear on *Grey's Anatomy* will soon become second nature to you, and pretty soon you'll be whipping out 50-cent words like a seasoned medical professional.

The Tale Behind the Terms

Medical terminology is made up of the terms that describe human anatomy and physiology (body organs, systems, and their functions), body locations, diseases, clinical, diagnostic imaging, and laboratory testing, together with clinical procedures, surgeries, and diagnoses.

It's important for every one of these things to have a specific name — just as it's important that you have your own unique name — because otherwise how would medical professionals be able to communicate clearly with one another? You might be able to visit your doctor and say, "I have a pain in my shoulder," and have him solve the mystery of what is causing that pain. But when your doc communicates that information to, say, a surgeon, it's crucial to be more specific. There are many working parts to your shoulder, after all, so you wouldn't want the surgeon to try and fix something that's not broken. When your doctor tells the surgeon the problem is with the rotator cuff, they are communicating much more clearly, and hopefully surgery and treatment will be a lot better.

The beauty of medical terminology is that it makes such vital communication more succinct and to-the-point. A medical term usually describes in one word a disease or condition that, under normal circumstances, would take several words to describe. *Appendectomy* is a one-word medical term to describe "surgical removal of the appendix." Now that saves you plenty of breath for more important things, like singing an aria or rooting for the Colts.

You can thank the Greeks and Romans for getting the ball rolling with regard to terminology, Hippocrates and Aristotle especially. Over 2,000 years ago, they saw the need for specific, descriptive medical language and began to create words that matched body parts and functions. Now, although you may secretly curse them as you study for your terminology final, you should also take the time to thank them for saving us a world of confusion.

The foundation of medical terminology is based in both Greek and Latin origin. The Greeks were the founders of modern medicine, but Latin is the basic source of medical terms. With origins in ancient Rome, Latin quickly made its way through the world, solidifying its rep as the language of choice for medicine and science. Building on guidance from the Greek and Latin origins, medical terms began to be professionalized in the mid-1800s. The first medical dictionary appeared in the 1830s shortly after the first edition of *Webster's American Dictionary of the English Language*.

Making Terminology Work for You

Thankfully, there are ways to wade through the quagmire of medical terms and figure out how to pronounce and use them like a champ. But you have to start at the beginning by breaking down the parts of each word and then deciphering its meaning. Or, to put it in a fancy-schmancy way, you should use etymology. *Etymology* helps you find the origin and historical development of a term. You can use etymology to decipher words with Latin and Greek origins, eponyms (words named after people), and acronyms (modern language terms that stand for longer phrases).

Back to those word parts that you'll break down. There are three you need to know:

- Roots/combining forms
- Prefixes
- Suffixes

Roots are the glue that holds all medical terms together. They are the basic form around which the final word is formed. A *combining form* is a combining vowel (usually *o* or *i*) plus the root word, usually with a prefix or suffix added. *Prefixes* appear at the beginning of a word and tell the how, why, where, when, how much, how many, position, direction, time, or status. The *suffix* always at the end of a word, usually indicates a procedure, a condition, or a disease. While the prefix gives us a clue into what to expect in a word's meaning, the suffix tells us what is happening with a specific body part or system. And, usually, it either entails what is wrong with you or the procedure used to diagnose or fix it.

Oh, but we're not done yet! In fact, the fun of medical terminology has just begun once you figure out the parts of each word. You can put words in plural form (which unfortunately involves way more than adding a simple *s*), find out how to pronounce them, and — the big payoff — use them in the real world.

The breaking down of words that you will learn in this book also helps you with pronunciation. With medical terminology, sounds are not always pronounced the same as in English, and there are no steadfast rules that a combination of specific letters will always be pronounced in the same way. One thing that helps in both the standard English and medical worlds, though, is to learn how to pronounce phonetically, by breaking up the word into smaller parts.

There is an old saying that the only constant is change. With medical terms, the same rule applies. A rule that might work for pronouncing one word might not come close to working for any other word. Be ready to be flexible, because what may seem familiar to you from everyday English might take on a whole new sound as a medical term. Once you can open your mind to all of the possibilities, you'll enter a whole new world of understanding terminology.

Building a Foundation of Vocabulary

Getting the basics of word formation and pronunciation down pat is the hard part. Once you can do that, you can move on to building your word vocabulary. Even though medical professionals like to joke that terminology is like a foreign language (sometimes, yes), don't throw this book out the window just yet. The good news is that you probably already know a lot of medical terms and you can use those to build up the rest of your newfound vocabulary. New terms become easier once you know the reasoning behind most medical terms.

Remember your grade school days when you used all kinds of little tricks to remember things like multiplication tables and the state capitals? The same principle applies to new medical terms. You can make lists of word parts, list words by similar sound, map words, or memorize terms by body system. And those are just a few ideas. Do whatever works for you, even if it's singing terms to the tune of "Sunrise, Sunset" in the shower. We promise not to tell.

In Terms of Anatomy

For our purposes in the land of medical terms, we can compare anatomy to the infrastructure of a building. The walls, floors, bricks, plaster, electrical system, plumbing, and so forth all help keep the building working for the people who inhabit it. Your body's anatomy is no different, which is why you are going to read about these particular terms first. Once you get the basics of what holds your body together, you can go on to find out about the physiological systems that make your body react to both internal and external circumstances.

First on our anatomy checklist is the skeletal system. This is your body's frame, much like the frame of a building. This system, along with its joints, works together with the muscles to give you the support and movement you need every day. The bony skeleton provides the jointed framework for the body, giving it shape. This framework protects vital organs from external injury and provides attachment points for muscles, ligaments, and tendons to make body movement possible.

Working together with the skeleton is the muscular system, in which several different major muscle groups work together. Made up of over 600 muscles and joints, this system is responsible for movement. The skeleton provides attachment points and support for muscles, but it is the muscle tissue's ability to extend and contract that makes movement possible.

Covering all this infrastructure is the integumentary system. Your skin, glands, nails, and hair work like the façade, or outside covering, of a building. They are the things people see when they look at you. The outside of your "building" often shows the world how healthy the rest of your body is. Healthy skin, along with accessory organs glands, hair, and nails, are the hallmarks of healthy insides, so care for them accordingly. Think of this as you would apartment shopping. If the outside of the building looks shoddy, would you want to move in?

Your sensory system is all of the "fun stuff" in your building. The windows, amenities, sound system, and dining facility all bring aesthetic delight to the building's inhabitants, and your senses work in a similar fashion. Your eyes are the windows to your world. Everything you see from your own face in the mirror each morning to the sight of the most beautiful sunset comes to you courtesy of those peepers. The smell of baking bread, the feel of a fine cashmere sweater, the taste of a great vintage wine, and the sound of a child's laughter are all made possible by your senses.

It may be hard to imagine that words can describe all of the amazing things your anatomy can do, but believe us when we say that it's all possible through terminology. And who knows? Perhaps there's a word out there that hasn't been created yet that you will coin using what you learn here.

All Systems Go

Once you get those basic working parts ingrained in your brain, you will move on to the physiology terminology. Physiology deals with the remaining body systems that help your fabulous body do its day-to-day work.

First up is the thing that keeps your blood pumping and your life moving forward each day: your heart. More specifically, the cardiovascular system. Your heart does not work in a vacuum. It has supporting players, namely your blood cells and vessels. These parts all work together to supply your body with fresh, clean, oxygenated blood.

Then there is the separate but complementary lymphatic system that works to flush your body of impurities. Most directly associated with immunity the lymphatic system works in the same context as the cardiovascular system due to the similar makeup of the system and the fact that, once cleaned by the lymph nodes, lymphatic fluid is released directly into the bloodstream. Lymph vessels are arranged in a similar pattern as the blood vessels.

Speaking of oxygenating your blood, think about how that oxygen finds its way into your body. You may not consciously think about it every day, but breathing makes it all possible. The body's trillions of cells need oxygen and must get rid of carbon monoxide, and this exchange of gases is accomplished by the respiratory system. External respiration is the repetitive, unconscious exchange of air between the lungs and the external environment.

You have to breathe, but you also have to eat, and eating is way more fun. Your good buddy the gastrointestinal system helps turn those tasty meals and treats into usable energy for your body. Also called the alimentary or digestive tract, this system provides a tube-like passage through a maze of organs and body cavities, beginning at the mouth, the food entrance into the body, and ending at the anus, where solid waste material exits the body. Voilá! Your delicious Chinese takeout magically turns into . . . well, you know.

Moving on, the complicated endocrine system maintains the chemical balance of the body. It does this by sending chemical messengers called hormones throughout the body via the bloodstream. Hormones regulate and control activity of specific cells or organs. Slowly released hormones control organs from a distance. Endocrine glands are located in different parts of the body. They are said to be ductless, because they have no duct system to transport their secretions. Instead, hormones are released directly into the bloodstream to regulate a variety of functions of body organs. One can stimulate growth, another matures sex organs, and yet another controls metabolism. Your body has both central and peripheral glands.

Even more complicated (are we having fun yet?) is the nervous system. Working like the body's built-in computer system, it is far more complex than your laptop. Messages from the brain are relayed via the spinal cord through nerve fibers that provide connections for incoming and outgoing data. The body has more than *ten billion* nerve cells whose function is to coordinate activities of the body. This system controls our voluntary activities as well as involuntary activities. We speak, hear, taste, see, think, move muscles, and have glands that secrete hormones. We respond to pain, danger, temperature, and touch. We have memory, association, and discrimination. These functions are only a small part of what the nervous system controls.

The nervous system is made up of the central nervous system (CNS), which includes the brain and spinal cord. The peripheral nervous system (PNS) is composed of cranial nerves (that extend from the brain) and spinal nerves (that extend from the spinal cord). The autonomic nervous system (ANS) controls and coordinates the functions of the body's vital organs, such as heartbeat and rate of breathing — functions we don't even think about.

Down Under Details

Speaking of things you don't usually think about, the urinary system is made up of the kidneys (two), ureters (also two), bladder, and urethra. This system's main function is to remove urea (the nitrogenous waste products of metabolism) from the bloodstream, and excrete it in urine from the body. Nitrogenous waste is difficult to excrete from the body. The main function of the urinary system is to remove urea from the bloodstream.

Urea is formed in the liver from ammonia. The bloodstream carries it (in the same manner as hormones and lymph) to the kidneys, where it passes with water, salts, and acids out of the bloodstream into the kidneys. The kidneys produce the urine that travels through each ureter into the bladder to be excreted via the urethra. Now that's a whole lot of information to impress your friends with at a dinner party. On second thought, maybe not.

When food and oxygen combine in cells to produce energy, the process is known as *catabolism*. In the process, food and oxygen are not destroyed, but small particles making up the food and oxygen are rearranged in a new combination, and the results are waste products. Waste in the form of gas (carbon dioxide) is removed from the body by exhaling through the lungs.

Think about how you were made. No, you weren't discovered under a cabbage leaf. Your mom and dad made you (see *Sex For Dummies* if you don't get our drift here) using their reproductive systems. In the male, it has two main functions: to produce spermatozoa, (the male reproductive cell) and to secrete testosterone (the male hormone) The reproductive organs, or gonads, are the testes. They are supported by accessory organs, ducts, glands, and supportive structures. The ducts include the epididymides (epididymis-singular) vas deferens, ejaculatory ducts, and the urethra. Glands include seminal vesicles, prostate, and bulbourethral glands (or Cowper's glands). The supporting structures include the penis, scrotum, and spermatic cords. That's a lot of moving parts.

The female reproductive system produces the female reproductive cell, or sex cell, secretes the hormones estrogen and progesterone, and provides, the conditions to establish a pregnancy, together with providing a safe place for the pregnancy to develop and grow. The gonads (ovaries in the female), together with the internal accessory organs consisting of the fallopian (uterine) tubes, uterus, vagina, external genitalia, and breasts (mammary glands) make up the reproductive system in the female. Reproduction is achieved by the union of the female reproductive cell, (an ovum) and the male reproductive cell, (a spermatozoon) (sperm for short), resulting in fertilization.

This is just a quick glance at the kinds of stuff you're going to learn about your body. Of course, the appropriate terms will be discussed in detail along with the simple biology background.

The Ultimate Resource: You

Before you crack open a frosty beverage and celebrate the fact that you've survived the first class of Terminology 101, take a few quick resources with you for the road. A listing of well-known term references, recall devices, and word-building activities will help you take your terminology show on the road and apply it to your own personal real-world situation.

The references mentioned in this book are some of the most well respected. Of course, there are thousands of online and print resources, most of which are reputable. Use your own good judgment when it comes to choosing one as your go-to source. In other words, it might be best to stay away from Joe Bob's House of Medical Terms.

As you go on this journey, remember that ultimately you are your own best source of tips and tricks. Maybe you're a flashcard aficionado. Perhaps you do best when you can visualize the term with the appropriate body system. Or maybe you like a good old pneumonic device like "*i* before *e* except after *c*." No matter how you choose to learn and recall these terms, do what is most comfortable and useful for you. You're the captain of this boat. Now, hoist the sail!

Coloring Books

FLASHCARD

USUALIZE = SYSTEM (LOCATION), PURPOSE

LISTINGS

WORD BUILDING ACTIVITIES

SPELL OUT WORDS TOO!

Chapter 2

Medical Terminology: The How and Why

*R*epeat after us: Context is a good thing.

You love context. Mmmmm, context. It is a good idea to get to know something about your subject matter before you dive head-first into studying it. This is particularly true with medical terminology because so much of the theory and history behind this topic shows up in the actual words and terms you will use every day.

Defining Medical Terminology

First, let's ponder what medical terminology is. It's a whole lot more than just medical words and phrases. Each word and each term is *organic*, meaning you can trace each part of the word back to a specific meaning. Cobbled together, these little meanings make up the overall meaning of the word.

Medical terminology is made up of terms that describe human anatomy and physiology (body organs, systems, and their functions), body locations, diseases, diagnostic imaging and laboratory testing, together with clinical procedures, surgeries, and diagnoses.

Why do we need medical terminology?

A medical term usually describes in one word a disease or condition that, under normal circumstances, would take several words to describe.

Sprechen Sie terminology?

Medical terminology is like a foreign language to most people. In fact, it operates exactly like a foreign language if you have never encountered it before. There are so many words that are difficult to pronounce and even more difficult to spell correctly. As such, medical terms sound strange, confusing, and sometimes overwhelming to the novice. They make no sense whatsoever. But as in a foreign country, you can't make out what is happening until you can speak the language.

Just as with practicing German (or any language, for that matter), you get the meaning of medical terms by breaking down each word into different parts:

✔ **Prefix:** Appears at the beginning of a word and tells the how, why, where, when, how much, how many, position, direction, time, or status.

✔ **Root word:** Specifies the body part to which the term refers.

✔ **Suffix:** Appears at the end of a word and indicates a procedure, condition, or disease

Those are the bare bones, basic parts of every medical term. Each prefix, root, and suffix has its own meaning, so it's your job to remember them and put the three meanings together into one greater word meaning. It can be tricky, though, so proceed carefully until you are confident of individual part meanings.

As with languages, things aren't always what they seem. For example, if we use tonsillitis and appendectomy, we see that the suffix -*itis* always means "inflammation," no matter what root word precedes it. Similarly, the suffix -*ectomy* always means "surgical removal of." So when switching suffixes, *appendicitis* means "inflammation of the appendix," and *tonsillectomy* means "surgical removal of the tonsils."

For example, consider two terms commonly known to most people. *Tonsillitis* is a one-word medical term to describe "inflammation of the tonsils," and *appendectomy* is a one-word medical term to describe "surgical removal of the appendix." It's much easier to use one word than a long, drawn-out phrase to describe these conditions, don't you think?

Using Medical Terminology in the Real World

The need or desire to learn medical terminology is not limited to the health-care professionals. For example, a firefighter has to relay information to paramedics, such as the condition of a burn victim being placed in an ambulance. A police officer must complete a written report after delivering a baby in the back seat of a car. Or closer to home, think about trying to understand when a doctor tells you that your child needs surgery, or why an aging parent needs to be placed in a long-term care facility.

And of course the best thing of all about medical terminology is that it allows you to convey the greatest quantity of information, with the least confusion and most precision, to anyone in the world. For example, saying someone has a badly broken wrist doesn't convey as much as saying someone has a Salter-Harris II fracture of the right digital radius with moderate lateral displacement and 28 degrees of upward angulation. Now who's the coolest kid in the clinic?

In theory and practice

You don't need prior knowledge of Greek and Latin or anatomy and physiology to build a medical vocabulary. But you do need to master the fundamentals, or the ABCs, so to speak, to be comfortable and confident with medical terminology.

You accomplish this by breaking down each word and identifying its parts (prefix, suffix, and root). A basic knowledge of the human anatomy helps, but more important is to know how each body system works independently and together with other systems. Knowing that helps the puzzle pieces fit into place more easily.

Mastering medical terms is much easier than you think. It is certainly easier than acquiring a whole new language from scratch. You already know words like *appendicitis* and *tonsillectomy*. New terms become easier once you know the reasoning behind most medical terms. Many terms are made up of interchangeable parts, used over and over again, in different combinations. Once you understand this, you will be well on your way to translating even the toughest medical terms — including terms you have never heard or seen before.

Your vocabulary will grow by leaps and bounds as you analyze medical terms, and you'll find that this will become the key to your success. Root words, suffixes, and prefixes make up the basis for all terms. As with your ABCs, once you have these mastered, the sky is the limit.

Writing it down

One thing that gives some people pause with medical terminology is spelling the words correctly. Again, defer to the rule of breaking down the word into parts. If you can spell each small prefix, root, or suffix and put them all together, then you can spell medical terms with ease.

One of the best ways to practice the spelling is, of course, to write it down.

Whether you are a list maker or prefer to draw maps, there is a way for you to incorporate writing terms as spelling and word-recognition practice. Some useful ideas for writing and recalling terms are

- ✔ Make lists of similar prefixes, roots, and suffixes based on what body system they are associated with.

- ✔ Make lists of prefixes, suffixes, and roots based on some other memorable moniker, such as sound similarity or similar meaning.

- ✔ Draw simple maps of each system and label body part terms.

- ✔ Use your body system map to identify diseases affecting each specific part. You can also use this technique to identify locations of specific procedures.

Building a medical vocabulary involves breaking down a word by identifying its prefix, suffix, and root word. The root word is the foundation or basic meaning of the word. It can appear with a prefix and suffix or between a prefix and suffix, as prefixes and suffixes never stand alone. They must be attached to a root word.

In this book we outline roots, suffixes, and prefixes and include the anatomy for each body system to help you to understand how everything fits together. When in doubt, look at the table of contents and check a specific body system's chapter.

Changes in Medical Terminology

Medical language is an entity unto itself and followed a historical development. Common medical vocabulary used today includes terms built from Greek and Latin word parts, some of which were used by Hippocrates and Aristotle more than 2,000 years ago. That's quite an extensive pedigree, and one that only continued to build as time flew by, right into the modern age.

One type of medical term is the *eponym*, a term named after the personal name of someone. An example would be Parkinson's disease, named after the English physician Dr. James Parkinson.

With the great advancements in medicine throughout the 20th century, medical language changed with the times and continues to do so today. Some words are discarded or considered obsolete, whereas others are changed, and new words are continually added.

Building on guidance from the Greek and Latin origins, medical terms began to be professionalized in the mid-1800s. *Dorland's Illustrated Medical Dictionary* was first published in 1890 as the *American Illustrated Medical Dictionary*, consisting of 770 pages, over 50 years after the first edition of *Webster's American Dictionary of the English Language*. Dr. William Alexander

Dorland was the editor, and when he died in 1956 the dictionaries were renamed to include his name, thus they are known today as *Dorland's Illustrated Medical Dictionary*. Electronic medical publishing took off during the 1980s thanks to advancements in database publishing and electronic storage. In the mid 1990s, medical dictionaries — most notably from Dorland's, Stedman's, and Taber's — became available in electronic form with many various editions and publications available on disk, CD-ROM, and via Internet downloading.

Now available in several formats including traditional print, CD-ROM, Web sites, databases, and even wall charts, medical dictionaries grow bigger with each new edition. Check out Chapter 24 for a list of great resources. The rapid increase in medical and scientific knowledge necessitates new medical vocabulary to describe it. Changes in medicine in the 20th century became apparent in the growing size of medical dictionaries. Knowledge about immunology, antibodies, allergies, and viruses was in the infancy stage in early editions of dictionaries.

It's Greek and Latin to Me

You can thank the two founding fathers of medical terminology for getting the ball rolling: Hippocrates and Aristotle. Hippocrates, considered the father of medicine, was a student, teacher, and great physician. Aristotle was a Greek philosopher and a physical scientist. He stressed observation and induction. His major studies were of comparative anatomy and physiology.

The Hippocratic Oath — an oath of professional behavior sworn by physicians beginning a medical career — is attributed to Hippocrates.

The Greeks were the founders of modern medicine, but Latin is the basic source of medical terms. With origins in ancient Rome and thanks to good, old-fashioned conquest, Latin quickly made its way through the world, solidifying its rep as the language of choice for medicine and science. You can still see evidence of Latin's influence in several languages, from English and French to Italian and Spanish.

When first confronted with medical terms, the average person is puzzled and often overwhelmed by the sometimes strange spelling and more so the pronunciation. This is understandable when approximately 75 percent of all medical terms are based on Latin or Greek terms. Most medical terms are derivatives of Latin and Greek, even though modern day changes are made to make the terms more comprehensive.

Look no further than the study of etymology to help you crack the code of medical terms. *Etymology* indicates the origin and historical development of a term. Some examples of etymology, or word history, include

✓ **Words with Latin origins:** *Femur*, for example, is a Latin term referring to a bone in the leg.

✓ **Words with Greek origins:** *Hemorrhage*, for example, is a word with Greek origin indicating a rapid, uncontrollable loss of blood.

✓ **Eponyms:** These are the words named after people, such as Parkinson's disease.

✓ **Acronyms:** These are modern language terms that stand for longer phrases such as *laser*, which stands for "light amplification by stimulated emission of radiation."

Etymologies were listed in early medical dictionaries, assuming the reader had studied languages and could read Greek or Latin. But gradually the Greek alphabet was cast aside when it was later recognized that few, aside from specialists, were actually studying ancient Greek.

Modernizing Medicine

With the advent of the medical dictionary, terminology came to the masses with full force. Today, medical terminology has evolved into modern applications from basic anatomy to include alternative, holistic, naturopathic, and complementary medicine. Other modern applications of medical terminology include (but are certainly not limited to):

✓ CAT scans

✓ DNA advancement

✓ Hundreds of new drugs on the market to assist or alleviate a multitude of ailments

✓ Investigative and diagnostic medicine

✓ Joint replacements and other surgical procedures

✓ Laparoscopic surgeries

✓ MRIs

✓ Organ transplants

✓ Stem-cell research

Today medical terminology is used and needed in any occupation that is remotely related to medicine and the normal functioning of the body.

To name a few careers involving the need for medical terminology:

- ✔ Athletic therapy
- ✔ Audiology
- ✔ Dentistry and dental hygiene
- ✔ Emergency medical services
- ✔ Exercise science
- ✔ Genetics
- ✔ Massage therapy
- ✔ Medical statistics
- ✔ Medical transcription
- ✔ Nutrition
- ✔ Occupational therapy
- ✔ Personal training
- ✔ Pharmacy
- ✔ Physical therapy
- ✔ Speech language
- ✔ Veterinary medicine

All these applications exist in addition to the obvious groups of healthcare professionals who use terminology in their day-to-day activities, including associates, the medical secretary in a doctor's office, the insurance claims adjuster, the compensation board adjudicator, the courtroom recorder . . . the list goes on and on. Even the proofreader of a local newspaper needs to know a little medical terminology in order to keep that medical news article free of spelling errors.

We see evidence of changes everywhere. A large percentage of surgeries are now done laparoscopically (using a fiberoptic scope), and new surgical instruments are introduced almost daily. Cosmetically, in addition to plastic surgery, there are now Botox and fat redistribution procedures. A drug reference book is obsolete almost from publication, as more and more new drugs flood the market. There is always a new cough medicine to try or allergy pill to take. With every new medical discovery comes the medical terminology that describes it. The study continues to evolve, even as you read this book.

The 31st Edition of *Dorland's Illustrated Medical Dictionary* advertises that it contains around 125,000 entries. The 29th edition of this same dictionary contains approximately 117,500 entries. That's an addition of 7,500 new words in just two editions!

Chapter 3

Introducing the Big Three: Prefixes, Roots, and Suffixes

*I*ntroducing the starting lineup for your medical terminology team! Whether you realize it or not, most words are made up of individual parts that contribute their own meaning. The big three — roots, prefixes, and suffixes — of medical terms all work together to clue you in to what that word means. Often, they tell you where it comes from, too.

Starting at center, you have the root. The *root* is the main part of the word, telling you in general the thing you are dealing with. The word root specifies the body part.

Playing forward is the prefix. A *prefix* appears at the beginning of a word and tells you more about the circumstances surrounding the meaning of the word.

The suffix would be the goalkeeper, to really stretch this metaphor. The *suffix* is always at the end of a word and, in the medical world, usually indicates a procedure, a condition, or a disease.

Almost every medical term can be broken down into some combination of prefixes, roots, and suffixes. Because they are the core of a word's meaning, the root words are great in number. There are many more roots than prefixes and suffixes put together.

Rooting Around for Answers

So what makes the root of a word so darned important? Maybe it's because the root lights the way to understanding the body system in question. The combining form, or word root, specifies the body part the word is either describing or associated with. Just by doing that, it helps rule out hundreds of other possibilities, allowing you to think only about a specific set of body parameters.

In this section are two big lists of all the important roots that can appear after any prefix or before any suffix. They divide into two categories: exterior root words, which describe the exterior of the body, and interior root words, which deal with — you guessed it — the inside. These are the big daddies, the glue that holds all medical terms together. Think of this section as one-stop shopping. If you can't find your root word here, you won't find it anywhere! We will not be undersold!

Exterior root words

Table 3-1 lists the root words and combining forms that pertain to the exterior of the body.

Table 3-1	Your Fabulous Façade: Exterior Root Words
Exterior Root	*What It Means*
Acr/o	Extremities
Anter/o	Front
Axill/o	Armpit, axilla
Blephar/o	Eyelid or eyelash
Brachi/o	Arm
Bucc/o	Cheek (on the face!)
Canth/o	Angle of the eyelids
Capit/o	Head
Carp/o	Wrist
Caud/o	Tail/downward
Cephal/o	Head
Cervic/o	Neck or cervix (neck of uterus)
Cheil/o, chil/o	Lip

Exterior Root	What It Means
Cheir/o, chir/o	Hand
Cili/o	Eyelash or eyelid, or small hair-like processes
Cor/e, cor/o	Pupil of eye
Derm/a, derm/o, dermat/o	Skin
Dors/i, dors/o	Back or posterior
Faci/o	Face
Gingiv/o	Gums in mouth
Gloss/o	Tongue
Gnath/o	Jaws
Inguin/o	Groin
Irid/o	Iris of eye
Labi/o	Lips
Lapar/o	Abdomen, loin, or flank
Later/o	Side
Lingu/o	Tongue
Mamm/a, mamm/o	Breast
Mast/o	Breast
Nas/o	Nose
Occipit/o	Back of the head
Ocul/o	Eye
Odont/o	Teeth
Omphal/o	Umbilicus
Onych/o	Nails
Ophthalm/o, ocul/o	Eyes
Optic/o, opt/o	Seeing, sight
Or/o	Mouth
Ot/o	Ear
Papill/o	Nipple
Pelv/o	Pelvis
Phall/o	Penis
Pil/o	Hair

(continued)

Table 3-1 *(continued)*

Exterior Root	What It Means
Pod/o	Foot
Rhin/o	Nose
Somat/o	Body
Steth/o	Chest
Stomat/o	Mouth
Tal/o	Ankle
Tars/o	Foot
Thorac/o	Chest / thorax
Trachel/o	Neck or necklike
Trich/o	Hair or hairlike
Ventr/i, ventr/o	Front of body

Interior root words

Now it's time to meet the movers and shakers that best define your inner self. Table 3-2 lists the root words and combining forms associated with the body's interior workings.

Table 3-2	Beautiful on the Inside: Interior Root Words
Interior Root	What It Means
Abdomin/o	Abdomen
Aden/o	Gland
Adren/o	Adrenal gland
Alveoli/o	Air sac
Angi/o	Vessel
Arteri/o	Artery
Arteriol/o	Arteriole
Athr/o	Joint
Atri/o	Atrium
Audi/o	Hearing
Balan/o	Glans penis
Bio-	Life

Interior Root	What It Means
Bronch/i, bronch/o	Bronchus
Bronchiol/o	Bronchiole
Carcin/o	Cancer
Cardi/o	Heart
Cellul/o	Cell
Cerebell/o	Cerebellum
Cerebr/i, cerebr/o	Cerebrum
Chol/e	Bile
Cholecyst/o	Gallbladder
Choledoch/o	Common bile duct
Chondr/i, chondr/o	Cartilage
Chrom/o	Color
Col/o	Colon
Colp/o	Vagina
Cost/o	Rib
Cry/o	Cold
Crypt/o	Hidden
Cutane/o	Skin
Cyan/o	Blue
Cysti, cyst/o	Bladder or cyst
Cyt/o	Cell
Dipl/o	Double, twice
Duoden/o	Duodenum
Encephal/o	Brain
Enter/o	Intestine
Episi/o	Vulva
Erythr/o	Red
Esophag/o	Esophagus
Fibr/o	Fibers
Galact/o	Milk
Gastr/o	Stomach
Glyc/o	Sugar
Gynec/o	Female

(continued)

Table 3-2 *(continued)*

Interior Root	What It Means
Hemat/o	Blood
Hepat/o, hepatic/o	Liver
Heter/o	Other, different
Hidr/o	Sweat
Hist/o, histi/o	Tissue
Hom/o, home/o	Same, alike
Hydr/o	Water, wet
Hyster/o	Uterus
Iatr/o	Treatment
Ile/o	Ileum (intestine)
Ili/o	Ilium (pelvic bone)
Intestin/o	Intestine
Jejun/o	Jejunum
Kerat/o	Cornea of eye, horny tissue
Lacrima	Tears
Laryng/o	Larynx
Leuk/o	White
Lipid/o	Fat
Lith/o	Stone (in gallbladder or kidney)
Lymph/o	Lymph vessels
Melan/o	Black
Men/o	Menses, menstruation
Mening/o	Meninges
Metr/a, metr/o	Uterus
My/o	Muscle
Myel/o	Bone marrow or spinal cord
Myring/o	Eardrum
Nat/o	Birth
Necr/o	Death
Nephr/o	Kidney
Neur/o	Nerve
Oophor/o	Ovary

Interior Root	What It Means
Orchid/o, orchi/o	Testis
Oss/eo, oss/i, ost/e, ost/eo	Bone
Palat/o	Roof of mouth
Path/o	Disease
Peritone/o	Peritoneum
Pharmac/o	Drug
Pharyng/o	Pharynx
Phleb/o	Vein
Phren/o	Diaphragm
Pleur/o	Pleura, rib (side)
Pneum/a, pneum/o	Lungs
Pneum/ato, pneum/ono	Lungs
Poli/o	Gray matter of nervous system
Proct/o	Rectum, anus
Pulmon/o	Lungs
Py/o	Pus
Pyel/o	Pelvis of kidney
Rect/o	Rectum
Ren/i, ren/o	Kidney
Sacr/o	Sacrum
Salping/o	Fallopian tube
Sarc/o	Flesh
Scapul/o	Scapula
Sept/o	Infection
Splen/o	Spleen
Spondyl/o	Vertebra
Stern/o	Sternum
Tend/o, ten/o	Tendon
Testicul/o	Testis
Therm/o	Heat
Thorac/o	Chest
Thym/o	Thymus
Thyr/o	Thyroid gland

(continued)

Table 3-2 *(continued)*

Interior Root	What It Means
Thyroid/o	Thyroid gland
Tonsill/o	Tonsils
Trache/o	Trachea
Tympan/o	Eardrum
Ur/e, ur/ea, ur/eo, urin/o, ur/o	Urine
Ureter/o	Ureter
Urethr/o	Urethra
Vas/o	Vas deferens
Vas/o, ven/o	Vein
Vesic/o	Bladder
Viscer/o	Viscera (internal organs)
Xanth/o	Red, redness
Xer/o	Dry

Copycats and opposites

Some prefixes might look very different, but have the same meaning. Here are some examples:

✔ *Anti-* and *contra-* mean against.

✔ *Dys-* and *mal-* mean bad or painful.

✔ *Hyper-*, *supra-*, and *epi-* all mean above.

✔ *Hypo-*, *sub-*, and *infra-* all mean below.

✔ *Intra-* and *endo-* mean within.

However, other, more troublesome prefixes mean the opposite of each other even though they look or sound similar. These are contentious prefixes:

✔ *Ab-* means away from (abduct), but *ad-* means toward.

✔ *Ante-*, *pre-*, and *pro-* mean before, but *post-* means after.

✔ *Hyper-*, *supra-*, and *epi-* mean above, but *hypo-*, *infra-*, and *sub-* mean below.

✔ *Macro-* means large, while *micro-* means small.

✔ *Tachy-* means fast, but *brady-* means slow.

✔ *Hyper-* also means excessive, yet *hypo-* also means deficient.

It's just semantics

Take a moment to digest what exactly is meant by the word *semantics*. *Semantics* is, quite simply, the study of meaning in communication.

Have you ever heard someone say, "Let's drill down to semantics"? What they probably meant was that they wanted to discuss the actual meaning of whatever it was you were discussing. So, remember that when you are trying to decipher the meaning of a medical term, you do, in fact, want to talk semantics.

The word *semantics* is derived from the Greek *semantikos*, meaning "significant."

This may be a book about medical terms, but we're talking morphemes here, not morphine. A *morpheme* is the smallest linguistic unit that has semantic meaning. For example, *un* means not, or opposite. So the next time you look at a two-letter prefix and think it's just window dressing, think again. Chances are it has plenty of important meaning.

Prefix as Precursor

Think of the prefix as the welcome wagon for a term. It invites you in, welcoming you to a whole new world. It tells you something about what you are going to find inside. Prefixes and suffixes are modifiers or adjectives that alter the meaning of the root word, in the same ways as regular English terms. A prefix appears at the beginning of a word and tells the how, why, where, when, how much, how many, position, direction, time, or status.

An easy word-building activity is to use the prefixes you know and draw connections to medical terms you are familiar with. For example, you probably know that *ultra-* means something is extra, or beyond its normal scope. And you're probably familiar with the word *ultrasound*, a procedure that provides — you guessed it — a look at your insides that is beyond the normal scope of visual exam. See? You're a medical terminology whiz already. Okay, maybe I'm exaggerating slightly.

You might recognize many of the prefixes associated with medical terminology, because they have similar meanings in regular, everyday vernacular. For example, the most basic prefix of *a-* means without, or not, in medical terminology, just as it does in any other word. If something is atypical, it is not typical. *Hemi-* means half, as in *hemisphere*. The moral of this story is that prefixes aren't just window dressing. They have a unique and specific goal, which is to tell the reader more about the circumstances surrounding the word's meaning.

Common Prefixes

You can read a lot more about prefixes in Chapter 6, but to whet your appetite Table 3-3 gives you a quick look at some of the most common prefixes that play a huge role in both common, everyday English and medical terminology.

Table 3-3	Preview of Important Prefixes
Prefix	*What It Means*
A-, an-	Lack of, without, not
Ante-	Before, in front of, or forward
Anti-	Opposing or against
Bi-	Double, two, twice, both
Co-, con-, com-	Together or with
De-	Down, or from
Di-	Twice or two
Extra-, extro-	Beyond, outside of, or outward
Hemi-, semi-	Half, half of
Hyper-	Above, excessive, beyond
Hyp-, hypo-	Below, beneath, deficient
Intro-	Into, or within
Macro-	Large
Micro-, micr-	Tiny, small
Post-	After, or following, behind
Pre-, pro-	In front of, before, preceding
Retro-	Behind, backward
Semi-	Half
Trans-	Through or across
Tri-	Three
Ultra-	Excessive, beyond

Suffixes: Final Thoughts

The suffix, always at the end of a word, usually indicates a procedure, a condition, or a disease. Whereas the prefix gives us a clue into what to expect in a word's meaning, the suffix pulls no punches and tells us what is happening with a specific body part or system. And, usually, it either entails what is wrong medically or indicates the procedure used to diagnose or fix it.

The scope of suffix meanings is extremely wide. Like prefixes, many of these have similar meanings in plain old, everyday English that you hear on the street. For example, the suffix *-meter* simply indicates an instrument used to measure something, just as it does in other fields of study. Geography, a term feared by many fifth graders the world over, ends with *-graphy* and means the process of recording. You'll meet several other forms of *-graphy* in our medical term discussions.

Table 3-4 gives you a preview of the delights that await you in Chapter 7.

Table 3-4	Summarizing Important Suffixes
Suffix	*What It Means*
-ac, -ic, -al, -ous, -tic	Related to, or pertaining to
-ate, -ize	Subject to, use
-ent, -er, -ist	Person, agent
-genic	Produced by
-gram	A written record
-graph	Instrument used to record
-ism	Condition or theory
-ologist	One who studies, specialist
-ology	Study of, process of study
-phobia	Morbid fear of or intolerance
-scope	Instrument used to visually examine

Chapter 4

Acronyms, Eponyms, Homonyms, Multiples, and Plurals — Oh My!

*A*fter you've got the basics under your belt, it's time to branch out. Really branch out — in multiple directions. You might think that in medical terminology, multiples and plurals work just like they do for regular words in the English language.

Psych!

Read on to find out about the wily world of medical multiples.

Pluralized medical terms would be pretty easy to comprehend and remember if all examples followed the same rules. The fun (fun?) of the English language is that there seem to be just as many words that do *not* follow the rules as ones that do. To see this, all you have to do is look to some basic examples from everyday conversation.

Wouldn't it be simple if the standard rule was to add an *s* to make a noun plural? One cat and one dog would then become two or more *cats* and *dogs*. Simple. How about one woman, one man, and one child? This pluralization becomes two or more *women*, *men*, and *children*. So much for simply adding the *s*.

For the most part, terms of Latin or Greek origin *do not* follow English rules when it comes to pluralizing. However, luckily for you, in modern current use it is becoming more and more acceptable for medical terms to be pluralized by the English method.

But first, let's take a quick look at three common kinds of common medical terminology: acronyms, eponyms, and homonyms.

Acronyms

An *acronym* is a word (or abbreviation) formed by the first letters or syllables of other words. Most acronyms are expressed in uppercase letters, but not always. For example, you might be familiar with the words *scuba* and *laser.* These terms are so well known that they have become acceptable as words in their own right. *Scuba* began life as an acronym for *self-contained underwater breathing apparatus. Laser* was an acronym for *light amplification by stimulated emission of radiation.* These two humble acronyms went on to greater glory as bona fide words.

There are, to put it mildly, many acronyms in medical terminology, some of which are common, some not so common. It is important to know the context in which they are used, because many are identical or sound similar, but have quite different meanings. Here are some common medical acronyms.

- ✔ **AMA:** American Medical Association
- ✔ **AMA:** Against medical advice
- ✔ **CAT:** Computerized axial tomography (scan)
- ✔ **CAT:** Children's apperception test
- ✔ **COPD:** Chronic obstructive pulmonary disease
- ✔ **COPE:** Chronic obstructive pulmonary emphysema
- ✔ **ECT:** Electroconvulsive therapy (shock therapy)
- ✔ **ECT:** Enteric-coated tablet
- ✔ **ECT:** Euglobulin clot test
- ✔ **MRI:** Magnetic resonance imaging
- ✔ **MRI:** Medical Research Institute
- ✔ **MRI:** Medical records information

As you can see, many acronyms look the same, but actually mean something different. Knowing the *context* in which an acronym is being used is very important. Many common acronyms can be misinterpreted.

A favorite acronym of many medical professionals is BM. If you have ever been a patient in hospital, the usual question always asked by the nurse is, "Have you had a BM today?" Of course, most people know the nurse is referring to a bowel movement, but BM also could mean basal metabolism, body mass, bone marrow, basement membrane, blood monocyte, breast milk, or Bachelor of Medicine. Face it — everyone loves a good BM joke.

Next on the tour of plural forms is the antonym, proving once and for all that opposites do attract. An *antonym* is a word that means the opposite of another word. Examples would be right/wrong, right/left, up/down, and front/back. With reference to medical terms, some prefixes can be paired as opposites. Table 4-1 lists some of the most popular.

Table 4-1	Medical Antonyms
Prefix	*What It Means*
Ab-	Moving away from (abduction)
Ad-	Drawing toward (adduction)
Anterior-	Front
Posterior-	Back
Bio-	Life
Necro-	Death
Brady-	Slow
Tachy-	Fast
Cephalo-	Head (upward)
Caudo-	Tail (downward)
Endo-	Within, inside
Exo-	Outside
Eu-	Normal, well
Dys-	Difficult, unwell
Hyper-	Above or excessive
Hypo-	Below or deficient
Leuko-	White
Melano-	Black
Pre-	Before or in front of
Post-	After or behind
Proximal-	Near (think proximity)
Distal-	Away from (think distance)
Superior-	Above
Inferior-	Below

Eponyms

Eponyms are an unusual and interesting facet of the plural world. An *eponym* is a person, place, or thing from which a person, place, or thing, gets (or is reputed to get) its name. For example, Romulus is the eponym of Rome. It can also refer to a person whose name is a synonym for something (from the Greek *eponymos*: *epi* [to] + *onyma* [name]).

In the medical field a disease, sign, operation, surgical instrument, syndrome, or test is often named after a certain physician, surgeon, scientist, or researcher — someone responsible for the creation, improvement, or research involved in its discovery.

In current usage, it is now acceptable to drop the possessive apostrophe from most eponyms, so either is acceptable. For example, you can use Alzheimer's or Alzheimer.

Here are some of the most popular medical eponyms:

- **Apgar score:** Named after Virginia Apgar, American anesthesiologist (1909–1974). A numbering expressing the condition of a newborn infant at 1 minute of age and again at 5 minutes.

- **Alzheimer's disease:** Named for Alois Alzheimer, a German neurologist (1864–1915). A progressive degenerative disease of the brain.

- **Cushing's syndrome:** Named for Harvey Williams Cushing, American surgeon (1869–1939). A complex of symptoms caused by hyperactivity of the adrenal cortex.

- **Down syndrome:** Named after John Haydon Down, English physician (1828–1896). A chromosomal disorder, also called trisomy 21, formerly called mongolism.

- **Gleason grade:** Named for Donald Gleason, American pathologist (1920–Present). A rating of prostate cancer assigning scores of 1–5 for degrees of primary and secondary growth.

- **Hodgkin's disease:** A form of malignant lymphoma. Named for Thomas Hodgkin, an English physician (1798–1866).

- **Homans' sign:** Named for John Homans, American surgeon (1877–1954). Pain on dorsiflexion of the foot; a sign of thrombosis of deep veins of the calf.

- **Ligament of Treitz:** Located in the intestinal tract. Named after Wenzel Treitz, a Czech physician (1819–1872).

✔ **Lyme disease:** A multisystemic disorder transmitted by ticks. Named after a place, Old Lyme, Connecticut, where the disease was first reported in 1975.

✔ **Peyronie's disease:** Named for Francois de la Peyronie, a French surgeon (1678–1747). It means a deformity or curvature of the penis caused by fibrous tissue within the tunica albuginea. When distortion of the penis is severe it causes erectile dysfunction or severe pain during intercourse.

✔ **Parkinson's disease:** Named for James Parkinson, English physician (1755–1824). A group of neurological disorders including tremors and muscular rigidity.

As you can see, most of those famous people are no longer with us. So you had a much better chance of having something named after you if you were born a hundred years ago.

Don't be afraid to learn more about eponyms. Many diseases, signs, syndromes, and tests are listed in a medical dictionary. Any name can be researched as most are cross-indexed in a good medical dictionary such as *Dorland's*.

Homonyms

Similar to the antonyms is the homonym. A *homonym* is a word that has the same pronunciation as another, but a different meaning, and in most cases a different spelling (from the Greek *homonymos*: homos [same] + *onyma* [name]. Some common English language homonyms would be meat and meet, peal and peel, bare and bear, feet and feat, or pain and pane. While the list could go on and on with everyday English words, there are a few true homonyms in medical terminology. Table 4-2 shows the most likely suspects.

Table 4-2	Medical Homonyms
Word	*What It Means*
Humerus	A long bone in the upper arm
Humorous	Funny
Ileum	A portion of the colon
Ilium	A part of the pelvic bone
Lice	A parasite

(continued)

Table 4-2 *(continued)*

Word	What It Means
Lyse	To break
Loop	An oval or circular ring, by bending
Loupe	Magnifying glass or lens
Mnemonic	To assist in remembering
Pneumonic	Pertaining to the lungs (the "p" is silent)
Mucus	Secretion of the mucous membranes
Mucous	Adjective form of mucus (resembling mucus)
Plane	Anatomic (imaginary) level
Plain	Not fancy (plain x-rays)
Plural	More than one
Pleural	Pertaining to the lung
Radical	Extreme or drastic
Radicle	A vessel's smallest branch
Venus	A planet
Venous	Pertaining to a vein

Deriving a Plural the Medical Way

As you read earlier in this chapter, medical plurals are a bit different from the standard, everyday English variety. Read on to familiarize yourself with the nuances of medical plural building.

Medical rules for forming plurals

Some rules for pluralizing medical terms are as follows, with examples of the rule and exceptions to the rule.

Medical Rule 1: Change the a ending to ae

In other words, *vertebra* becomes *vertebrae*.

By adding the *e* to the plural, the "aah" sound ending pronunciation becomes "eh."

- Axilla, axillae
- Bursa, bursae
- Conjunctiva, conjunctivae
- Scapula, scapulae
- Sclera, sclerae

Medical Rule 2: Change the um ending to a
The *a* at the end is pronounced "aah."

- Acetabulum, acetabula
- Antrum, antra
- Atrium, atria
- Bacterium, bacteria
- Diverticulum, diverticula
- Labium, labia
- Medium, media

Medical Rule 3: Change the us ending to i
The *i* at the end is pronounced "eye."

- Alveolus, alveoli
- Bronchus, bronchi
- Coccus, cocci
- Embolus, emboli
- Fungus, fungi
- Glomerulus, glomeruli
- Meniscus, menisci
- Syllabus, syllabi (but syllabuses is also acceptable)

The exceptions to this rule include the following:

- Corpus, corpora
- Meatus, meatus (stays the same)
- Plexus, plexuses
- Viscus, viscera

Medical Rule 4: Change the is ending to es

The *es* is pronounced "eez."

- ✔ Analysis, analyses
- ✔ Diagnosis, diagnoses
- ✔ Exostosis, exostoses
- ✔ Metastasis, metastases
- ✔ Prognosis, prognoses
- ✔ Testis, testes

The exceptions to this rule are

- ✔ Epididymis, epididymides
- ✔ Femoris, femora
- ✔ Iris, irides

Medical Rule 5: Change the ma or oma ending to mata

- ✔ Carcinoma, carcinomata
- ✔ Condyloma, condylomata
- ✔ Fibroma, fibromata
- ✔ Leiomyoma, leiomyomata

In the Rule 5 examples, the English plural is also acceptable: condylomas, carcinomas, leiomyomas, and fibromas.

Medical Rule 6: When a term ends in yx, ax, or ix, change the x to c and add es

- ✔ Appendix, appendices
- ✔ Calyx, calyces
- ✔ Calix, calices (Strange but true, both are correct)
- ✔ Thorax, thoraces

Medical Rule 7: When a term ends in nx, change the x to g and add es

- ✔ Larynx, larynges
- ✔ Phalanx, phalanges

Medical Rule 8: For Latin medical terms that consist of a noun and adjective, pluralize both terms

- ✔ Condyloma acuminatum, condylomata acuminata
- ✔ Placenta previa, placentae previae
- ✔ Verruca vulgaris, verrucae vulgares

There are (of course!) some exceptions to all of these rules:

- ✔ Cornu, cornua
- ✔ Pons, pontes
- ✔ Vas, vasa

English rules of forming plurals

Many medical terms apply basic English rules for forming plurals. Thank goodness! You will no doubt recognize many of these common English language plural rules.

English Rule 1: Add an s

- ✔ Bronchoscope, bronchoscopes
- ✔ Disease, diseases
- ✔ Endoscope, endoscopes
- ✔ Finger, fingers
- ✔ Vein, veins

English Rule 2: When a term ends in s, x, ch, or sh, add es

- ✔ Crutch, crutches
- ✔ Distress, distresses
- ✔ Patch, patches
- ✔ Stress, stresses

English Rule 3: When a term ends in y after a consonant, change the y to i and add es

- ✔ Artery, arteries
- ✔ Bronchoscopy, bronchoscopies

✔ Endoscopy, endoscopies

✔ Ovary, ovaries

✔ Therapy, therapies

English Rule 4: When a term ends in o after a consonant, add nes

✔ Comedo, comedones

Exceptions:

✔ Embryo, embryos

✔ Placebo, placebos

When in doubt use a dictionary — it would be impossible to list all exceptions to all the rules.

Welcome to the Peanut Gallery: More Exceptions to the Plural Rules

Medical professionals, including physicians, clinicians, and pharmacists, often use measurements and their abbreviations to convey important information. In regard to *multiples*, the plural has no place in measurement abbreviations if coupled with a number value.

For example, the phrase "The incision was several centimeters long" is acceptable because it is a vague, not an exact amount. But if coupled with a number value and a measurement abbreviation, it then becomes, "The incision was 7 cm long." The measurement abbreviation *cm* is always used with a number value and is always singular. It is never pluralized as *cms*, as the number value provides the clue that someone is talking about more than one centimeter.

Another example of common measurement is the tablespoon. When made plural, this word becomes *tablespoons*. Used with a specific number value, it becomes *2 tablespoons*. When abbreviated, it is always *2 tbsp.*, not *2 tbsps*.

Abbreviation of measurement with numbers is always left singular.

Single-digit numbers are made plural by adding an *'s*. For example, "Several 4 × 4's were needed to build the porch" And "The patient was asked to count by 7's." However, no apostrophe is used to form the plural of multiple-digit numbers, including years. "He is in his early 20s" (not his 20's). "She was born in the 1950s" (not the 1950's). Get the picture?

Similarly, to pluralize uppercase abbreviations or acronyms, use a lowercase *s* without an apostrophe. Some medical examples include

- ✔ CVA, CVAs
- ✔ EEG, EEGs
- ✔ WBC, WBCs

But if the abbreviation is expressed in lowercase, then an 's (with the apostrophe) is added to pluralize.

- ✔ rbc's, not rbcs
- ✔ RBCs, not RBC's

The real culprits in medical terminology are what are called the *sound-alikes*. These words are pronounced almost the same, but with a different spelling and often a very different meaning. Not knowing the difference can get you into a lot of trouble and can cause a great deal of confusion. Table 4-3 shows several examples.

Table 4-3	Troublesome Sound-Alikes
Word	*What It Means*
Ablation	Surgical removal
Oblation	A religious offering
Access	A means of approaching
Axis	Center
Afferent	Towards the center
Efferent	Away from the center
Anecdote	A funny story
Antidote	A remedy to treat poisoning
Apparent	Clear, obvious
Abberant	Off course, abnormal
Aural	Pertains to the ear
oral	Pertains to the mouth
Callous	Hard like a callus, hardened thinking
Callus	Hardened area of skin
Cecal	Pertains to the cecum
Fecal	Pertains to feces

(continued)

Table 4-3 *(continued)*

Word	What It Means
CNS	Central nervous system (abbreviation)
C&S	Culture and sensitivity (lab test)
Discreet	Reserved or private
Discrete	Separate
Dysphagia	Difficulty eating or swallowing
Dysphasia	Difficulty speaking
Effusion	Escape of fluid into tissue
Infusion	To introduce fluid into vein or tissue
Ethanol	Alcohol
Ethenyl	Vinyl
Graft	Tissue implant from one area to another
Graph	Diagram
Joule	Energy
Jowl	Flesh on the jaw
Labial	Lip-like
Labile	Unstable
Liver	Body organ
Livor	Discoloration of skin after death
Palpation	To feel with the fingers
Palpitation	Rapid heartbeat
Perfusion	Pouring over or through
Profusion	Abundant, much
Protrusion	Jutting out
Perineal	Referring to the perineum (genital area)
Peritoneal	Referring to the peritoneum (membrane in abdominal, pelvic cavities)
Peroneal	Vein in the leg
Pleuritis	Inflammation of the pleura of the lung
Pruritus	Itching
Precede	To come before

Word	What It Means
Proceed	To carry on or continue
Prostatic	Pertaining to the prostate gland
Prosthetic	An artificial device replacing a body part
Scleroderma	Hardening of the skin
Scleredema	Swelling of the face
Shoddy	Poor quality of work
Shotty	Resembles buckshot

Perineal, *peritoneal*, and *peroneal* are famous screw-ups among many in the medical field. Don't join the crowd!

I before E: Memorization techniques

Everyone has their own favorite way of remembering words. The best thing to do is play around and find the memorization method that works best for you. Try some of these on for size:

✔ **Alphabetical order:** List prefixes, suffixes, or roots in alphabetical order to memorize.

✔ **Flashcards:** Use any connections you want to create your own flashcards.

✔ **Group words in similar body systems:** Tackle your list by system, recalling and memorizing one at a time, such as cardio-vascular, muscular, urinary, and so on.

✔ **Memorize by meaning:** Try grouping words with similar meanings.

✔ **Memorize by similar prefix or suffix:** If prefixes or suffixes are close in sound, spelling, or meaning, try lumping them together and memorizing in chunks.

✔ **Mnemonic devices:** Remember "I before E, except after C"? See if you can create your own mnemonic devices for medical terms.

✔ **Timed self-quizzes:** When you feel you've mastered a group of words, create your own self-quizzes (or find some online) and time yourself.

Then we have a handful of terms that never change, no matter what. Consider putting these at the top of your memorization to-do list.

✔ **Some words are always plural:** herpes and ascites.

✔ **Some are always singular:** adnexa or genitalia (not adnexae or genitaliae).

✔ **Some remain the same whether singular or plural:** biceps, triceps, forceps, and scissors.

Chapter 5

Say What? Pronunciation and Usage

In This Chapter

▶ Simplifying your pronunciation methods.

▶ Distinguishing prefix sounds from suffix sounds.

▶ Applying pronunciation tips to everyday usage and word building.

*I*f you read Chapter 4, you now have a better idea of how medical terms are formed. But unless you work on the set of a silent medical movie, you're going to have to learn how to pronounce these words. Even the Hollywood hotshots who rush around the sets of *ER* and *Grey's Anatomy* have to learn how to say medical terms, and are paid well to do it convincingly. Though you may not net seven figures for shouting, "Get an MRI of this man's duodenum and jejunum, stat!" you will fit right in with your medical counterparts by knowing the correct way to pronounce medical terms.

Hooked on Phonics

With medical terminology, sounds are not always pronounced the same as in your everyday English pronunciation, and there are not even steadfast rules that a combination of specific letters will always be pronounced in the same way. One thing that helps in both the standard English and medical worlds, though, is to learn how to pronounce *phonetically* — by breaking up the word into smaller parts.

The variety of possible letters and sound combinations can make — or at least can seem to make — medical terms difficult to pronounce, especially if you've never seen or heard the term before. What may seem familiar to you from everyday English might take on a whole new sound in a med term.

We can't repeat this enough: By breaking the word down into basic parts — prefix, root, and suffix — you can simplify the task of pronunciation.

Take a closer look at the prefixes and the combining forms or root words when you start vocalizing the terms you know. You will find that by adding a variety of suffixes, not only does the prefix and suffix change the definition of the term, more importantly, in many instances it changes the way the term is pronounced. What does this mean for you? It means dive into this book and start memorizing! This in itself is a difficult task, but thankfully, there are some basic rules and tips that you can apply to help you along the way.

Pronouncing Common Prefixes and Beginning Sounds

You have to start somewhere, so why not at the beginning? Because many medical terms start with an odd (to the English speaker's eye) combination of letters, the pronunciation isn't always obvious. Some letters are silent that aren't normally in the English language, whereas some letters take on a whole new sound. Clear as mud, right? Let's take a look at some common rules to help clarify things a bit.

The sound of silence

Terms beginning with the letters *ps* are pronounced with an "s" sound. The *p* is silent, as it usually is when it appears at the beginning of a medical word.

Remember that the "pee" is silent — like it is in a swimming pool.

Examples:

> Psychiatry: (sigh-KIYA-tree)
>
> Psychology: (sigh-CALL-ogy)

Terms beginning with *pn* are pronounced only with the "n" sound. Again, the *p* is silent.

Example:

> Pneumonia: (new-MOAN-ia)

Terms beginning with *pt* work exactly the same. Once again, the *p* is silent.

Example:

Ptosis: (TOE-sis)

Terms beginning with *ch* often take on the hard consonant sound like a "k."

Examples:

Chronic: (KRON-ic)

Chromatin: (KROME-a-tin)

Terms beginning with *c* or *g* can take on sound of "s" or "j" if they come before *e*, *i*, or *y*.

Examples:

Cycle: (SIGH-cull

Cytoplasm: (SIGH-toe-plazm)

Genetic: (JEN-etic)

Giant: (J-EYE-unt)

But *c* and *g* have a hard sound before other letters.

Examples:

Cast: (CA-st)

Cardiac: (CARD-iak)

Gastric: (GAS-trick)

Gonads: (GO-nadz)

From your ear to the dictionary

That's a pretty good start, but now it's time to throw a wild card into the mix. What if you cannot see the term, but only hear it? Could you find it in a medical dictionary? Some good, old-fashioned memorization rules will help you recall those hard-to-pronounce beginnings.

If it begins with an "s" sound, it could begin with *c*, *ps*, or *s*:

Cytology: (sigh-TOL-oh-jee)

Psychiatrist: (sigh-KIY-a-trist)

Serology: (sir-ROL-oh-jee)

If it begins with a "z" sound, it could begin with *x* or *z*:

> Xeroderma: (zero-DER-mah)
>
> Zygote: (z-eye-GOAT)

If it begins with an "f" sound, it could begin with *f* or *p*:

> Flatus: (FLAY-tus)
>
> Phlegm: (FLEM — also note the silent *g* before *m*)

If it begins with a "j" sound, it could be *g* or *j*:

> Gingivitis: (JIN-jih-VIT-is)
>
> Jaundice: (JOHN-dis)

If it begins with a "k" sound, it could be *c*, *ch*, or *k*:

> Crepitus: (KREP-i-tus)
>
> Cholera: (CALL-er-ah)
>
> Kyphosis: (kie-FOE-sis)

Pronouncing Common Suffixes and Endings

You're not out of the woods yet. One might think that pronouncing the endings of words is fairly self-explanatory. But again, medical terminology is kind of like the curve ball of modern language. As such, letters don't always sound like what they look like. This section lists some things to remember about saying word endings.

For terms ending in *i* (usually to form a plural), the *i* is always pronounced "eye."

Examples:

> Glomerulus, glomeruli: (glom-MERUL-EYE)
>
> Radius, radii: (raid-ee-EYE)

Terms ending in *ae* (again often plurals) are pronounced "ee."

Example:

Vertebra, vertebrae: (VERT-e-bray)

In terms ending in *es* (you guessed it — often plurals), the *es* is pronounced as if it were a separate syllable.

Examples:

Naris, nares: (nar-EEZ)

Testis, testes: (test-EEZ)

Pronouncing Common Combinations

Now that you have established a few pronunciation rules, consider what happens to the pronunciation of a term when we combine a prefix with a root word or combining form, together with a suffix, and often a combining vowel. The combinations are endless.

Keep a few simple explanations in mind before you start combining word parts. To review:

- **Prefix:** Always at the beginning of a term. Modifies the word root that it precedes. It almost always indicates a location, number, time or period of time, or status.

- **Word root/combining form:** Usually indicates a body part, such as *cardi/o* for heart, *gastr/o* for stomach, and *neur/o* for nerve.

- **Suffix:** Appears at the end of a medical term. Usually, though not always, indicates a condition, procedure, disorder, or disease.

A *combining vowel* can be used to change the spelling of a term, making the pronunciation easier. A combining vowel is *not* used when the suffix begins with a vowel as this would make pronunciation difficult. A combining vowel is only used when the suffix begins with a consonant. For example, *gastr/o* pertains to the stomach. Adding the suffix *-itis*, meaning inflammation, results in the term *gastritis* (GAS-TRY-tis). If the combining vowel *o* were not removed, the result would be *gastroitis* creating a double vowel and a word more difficult to pronounce (GAS-TRO-it-is).

Putting It All Together

You've got all the tools, now you just need to use them to build your pronunciation skills. To do that, you have to get brave and start adding all of the word parts together. A long medical term must be broken up into the word parts in order to arrive at a definition and a pronunciation. You can do this in two ways.

Some people like to look at the suffix first to determine if the term is a condition, a procedure, disorder, or disease. Once the suffix is defined, you can then move to the beginning of the word to define the prefix, if there is one, and the word root. This method is preferred by many people just getting their feet wet in the world of medical terms.

Others prefer to tackle the term from the beginning, establishing a meaning for the prefix first, then moving to the word root, and to the suffix last of all.

The pronunciation of a word can sometimes change when you take some prefixes, couple them with root words, and add vowels and suffixes. Following are some examples:

- **Euthyroid (YOU-thyroid):** The prefix *eu* means normal. Before thyroid, it means that the thyroid is normal.

- **Febrile (FEB-ril):** Means to have a fever. Add the prefix *a,* which means being away from or without, and the word becomes *afebrile* (ay-FEB-ril), meaning without a fever.

- **Hypertension (high-per-TEN-shun):** High blood pressure

- **Hypotension (high-poh-TEN-shun):** Low blood pressure. Though there is not much difference in the pronunciation of hypertension and hypotension, and one means the opposite of the other, it is important to hear — and see — the different spelling of the prefix application.

- **Oliguria (ol-ig-YOUR-ee-ah):** Scanty or infrequent urination

- **Polyuria (pol-ee-YOUR-ee-ah):** Excessive or frequent urination

Suffixes can also affect the pronunciation of a word. Different suffixes can mean different pronunciations, particularly in respect to colors. Check out these two combinations and how the pronunciation and meaning change with altered suffixes:

- **Erythrocytes (eh-RITH-roh-sites):** Red blood cells

- **Erythrocytosis (eh-RITH-ROH-sigh-TOE-sis):** Having increased erythrocytes

- **Melanosis (mel-ah-NO-sis):** Unusual black pigmentation

- **Melanocytes (mel-ah-no-SITES):** Pigmentation cell in the skin layer

Terminology treasure hunting in the dictionary

It is important to remember that every medical term you see or hear may not appear in a medical dictionary as it is commonly spelled or pronounced. With so many root words, prefixes, and suffixes, the possible combinations would be endless, and the medical dictionary would become a set of encyclopedias. So when trying to find a term in a medical dictionary, you might have to look under the root word first and the prefix and suffix separately. Most commonly used terms are now listed alphabetically, but just because you can't find a term in the dictionary right away doesn't mean it doesn't exist. It just means you might have to piece together your own definition.

Even the more grounded basis of a word, the root or combining form, can change the way we say and see words. The combining vowel, in particular, can change the meaning and pronunciation:

- ✔ **Neuritis (new-RYE-tis):** Inflammation of a nerve (neur/o)

- ✔ **Neuropathy (new-OP-a-thee):** A condition of a nerve

- ✔ **Neuroplasty (NEW-row-PLAS-tee):** Surgical repair of a nerve

What Condition Your Condition Is In

Pronouncing terms for conditions can be easy if you familiarize yourself first with the root word of the condition, and then with the suffix. Let's use the simple, everyday stomach ailment as an example. By first pronouncing the root word, then adding different suffixes, you can up your vocabulary by a few points:

- ✔ **Gastro (gas-troh):** Stomach

- ✔ **Gastritis (gas-TRY-tis):** Inflammation of the stomach (-itis)

- ✔ **Gastrodynia (gas-troh-DYNEee-ah):** A pain in the stomach (-dynia)

- ✔ **Gastropathy (gas-TROP-a-thee):** A stomach condition (-pathy)

On the other hand, you can grow your condition vocabulary and usage skills by applying the suffix to a variety of roots:

- ✔ **Cardiomegaly (kar-dee-oh-MEG-ah-lee):** Enlargement of the heart

- ✔ **Hepatosplenomegaly (he-PATO-splen-oh-MEG-ah-lee):** Enlargement of the liver and the spleen (*splen/o* for spleen) and *hepat/o* for liver

- ✔ **-megaly (MEG-ah-lee):** Enlargement of

- ✔ **Splenomegaly (splen-oh-MEG-ah-lee):** Enlargement of the spleen

Suffering Suffixes

Suffixes play the most major role in the different ways procedural terms are spelled and pronounced. Lucky for you, there is a short list of very common suffixes that pertain to procedures. So, again, make the acquaintance of a short list of word parts and you get a world of words in return.

Here are some of the suffixes pertaining to procedures that create changes in pronunciation:

- **-centesis:** A surgical puncture to withdraw or aspirate fluid
- **-ectomy:** Surgical removal of
- **-otomy:** Surgical incision or cutting into
- **-ostomy:** Surgical creation of an artificial opening
- **-plasty:** Surgical repair
- **-scope:** An instrument used for visual examination
- **-scopy:** To see, or a visual examination
- **-gram:** Resulting record or picture
- **-graphy:** The process of recording a record or picture

Using those suffixes, watch the change in pronunciation depending on the suffix that is used:

- **Abdominocentesis (ab-DOM-ino-sen-TEE-sis):** Surgical puncture of the abdominal cavity
- **Abdominoplasty (ab-dom-ino-PLAST-ee):** Surgical repair of the abdomen
- **Bronchoscope (BRONK-o-scope):** Instrument used to examine bronchus
- **Bronchoscopy (bronk-OS-oh-pee):** Visual examination of bronchus using a bronchoscope
- **Cardiogram (CARD-ee-oh-gram):** Film produced by a cardiography
- **Cardiography (car-dee-OG-rah-fee):** Process of recording heart activity
- **Colostomy (koh-LOST-oh-me):** Surgical creation of an opening in the colon
- **Colotomy (kol-LOST-oh-me):** Surgical cutting into the colon
- **Endoscope (ENDO-scope):** Instrument used for internal visual examination
- **Endoscopy (en-DOS-koh-pee):** Visual examination using an endoscope

✔ **Mammogram (MAMM-oh-gram):** Resulting record of a mammography

✔ **Mammography (mamm-OG-rah-fee):** Process of examining breasts

✔ **Mammoplasty (mamm-oh-PLAS-tee):** Surgical repair to the breast

✔ **Oophoritis (ou-for-EYE-tis):** Inflammation of an ovary

✔ **Oophorectomy (ou-ou-for-ECT-om-ee):** Surgical removal of an ovary

✔ **Salpingectomy (sal-pin-JECT-oh-me):** Surgical removal of a fallopian tube

✔ **Salpingogram (sal-PIN-joe-gram):** Resulting record from salpingography

✔ **Salpingography (sal-pinj-OG-rah-fee):** Procedure to examine fallopian tube

Some of the examples here demonstrate how the pronunciation of a medical word can change just by adding *gram* versus *graphy* or *ectomy* versus *otomy*. Something as small as a one-letter change can change the sound and meaning entirely. Take *scope* versus *scopy*. One letter difference changes an instrument into an examination, and more importantly, changes the pronunciation even more.

So, practice your pronunciation. Say the terms out loud and get the emphasis on the right syllable! (SILL-ab-el!)

And now for the grand finale

So what, you ask, is the craziest medical term to pronounce? What can I wow my friends with at cocktail parties and class reunions? What would make even the technical advisors of *ER* shudder in delight?

Try these two 25-cent words on for size:

✔ **Salpingo-oophorectomy (sal-PING-oh/ou-ou-for-ECT-om-ee):** Surgical removal of an ovary and tube

✔ **Oophorosalpingectomy (OU-OU-for-oh-sal-pin-GECT-om-ee):** Also meaning surgical removal of an ovary and tube

Part II

Mapping Words and Bodies

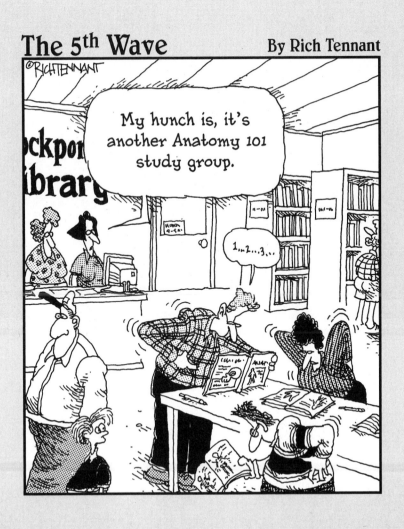

In this part . . .

Bring on the meaty basics of this book! Chapters 6 and 7 show you the possibilities of prefixes and suffixes. Chapter 8 shows you how to recognize words on your own terms. Chapter 9 teaches you how to break words down to make better sense of them. And Chapters 10 and 11 give you a more in-depth picture of the body and its systems, organs, and cavities.

Chapter 6

As It Was in the Beginning: Prefixes

- -

- -

*Y*ou first met your new friends, the prefixes, in Chapter 3. To recap: *Prefixes* show up at the beginning of a word and tell the how, why, where, when, how much, how many, position, direction, time, or status.

Prefixes have a very important job: They act as modifiers or adjectives, altering the meaning of the root word of the medical term. Though you will see in this chapter some new and unfamiliar prefixes that only exist in the medical world, for the most part medical prefixes work just like any other prefix in the English language.

Common Prefixes

Keep the other word part functions in mind when dealing with prefixes. The *combining form* or *root*, as explained in Chapter 3, specifies the body part. The *suffix*, always at the end of a word, usually indicates a procedure, condition, or disease. When all three work together, they make one powerful word.

First things first: Let's take a look at the most common prefixes in simple, easy-to-memorize alphabetical order. Later in the chapter we go over how these prefixes fit into everyday medical life and language.

A–E prefixes

- **A-, an-:** Lack of, without, not
- **Ab-:** Away from, take away
- **Ad-:** Towards or to, near
- **Ambi-, ambo-:** Both
- **Amphi-:** Double, both sides
- **Ana-:** Up, apart
- **Ante-:** Before, in front of, or forward
- **Anti-:** Opposing or against
- **Ap-, apo-:** Separated or derived from
- **Aut-, auto-:** Self, by yourself
- **Bi-:** Double, two, twice, both
- **Brady-:** Slow; most often refers to heart rhythm/rate
- **Brachy-:** Short
- **Cata-:** Lower, down, against
- **Circum-:** Around
- **Co-, con-, com-:** Together or with
- **Contra-:** Against or opposed to
- **De-:** Down or from
- **Di-:** Twice or two
- **Dia-:** Through, apart, across, between
- **Dis-:** Apart from or free from
- **Dys-:** Bad, painful, difficult
- **E-, ec-, ex-:** From, away from, out of
- **Ect-, exo-, ecto-:** Outside, outer, on
- **Em-, en-:** In
- **End-, endo-, ent-, ento-:** Within or inner
- **Epi-, ep-:** Upon, over, or on
- **Eu-:** Normal
- **Extra-, extro-:** Beyond, outside of, or outward

Kissing cousins: Different names, same meanings

Some prefixes look totally different, but have the exact same meaning. Check out these proxy prefixes:

Hyper-, supra- and *epi-* all mean "above."

Anti- and *contra-* mean "against."

Dys- and *mal-* both mean "bad" or "painful."

Hypo-, sub-, and *infra-* all mean "below."

Intra- and *endo-* mean "within."

Be on the lookout for prefixes that sound similar, but mean slightly different things, such as *ab-* and *ad-, ambi-* and *amphi-*, and *dis-* and *dys-*.

F–J prefixes

- ✔ **Hemi-, semi-:** Half, half of
- ✔ **Hyper-:** Above, excessive, beyond
- ✔ **Hyp-, hypo-:** Below, beneath, deficient
- ✔ **Im-, in-:** Into, in, within
- ✔ **Infra-:** Below or beneath
- ✔ **Inter-:** Between
- ✔ **Intra-:** Within, inside

    Infra-, inter-, and *intra-* are always mixed up and used inappropriately.

- ✔ **Intro-:** Into or within

K–O prefixes

- ✔ **Macro-:** Large
- ✔ **Mal-:** Bad
- ✔ **Mes-, meso-:** Middle
- ✔ **Meta-:** Beyond or changing
- ✔ **Micro-, micr-:** Tiny, small
- ✔ **Mono-, uni-:** One

- **Mult-, multi-:** Many, multiple
- **Neo-:** New or recent
- **Oligo-:** Scanty

 If you can't recall the meaning of a prefix, try putting into everyday English context. For example, you might remember the meaning of *macro-* by thinking about the word *macroeconomics*, which is about economics on a large scale.

P–Z prefixes

- **Pan-:** All
- **Para-:** Beyond, beside, or after
- **Per-:** Through
- **Peri-:** Around
- **Poly-:** Many, excessive
- **Post-:** After or following, behind
- **Pre-, pro-:** In front of, before, preceding
- **Presby-:** Old age
- **Pseudo-:** False
- **Quadri-:** Four
- **Re-:** Backward or again
- **Retro-:** Behind, backward
- **Semi-:** Half
- **Sub-:** Under or beneath
- **Super-, supra-:** Above, excessive, superior
- **Sym-, syn-:** With or together
- **Tachy-:** Rapid or fast
- **Trans-:** Through or across
- **Tri-:** Three
- **Ultra-:** Excessive, beyond

Not even close: Opposite prefixes

Some prefixes mean the opposite of each other:

Ab- means "away from" (*abduct*), but *ad-* means "toward."

Ante-, pre-, and *pro-* all mean "before," but *post-* means "after."

Hyper-, supra-, and *epi-* mean "above," but *hypo-, infra-,* and *sub-* mean "below."

Tachy- means "fast," whereas *brady-* means "slow."

Macro- means "large," whereas *micro-* means "small."

Hyper- means "excessive," but *hypo-* means "deficient."

Matching Prefixes to Situations

The next step in prefixes is applying them to the words we use every day in medical terminology. Keep in mind that the following is not by any stretch the end-all, be-all, conclusive list of medical words, but it's a nice sampling of prefixes at work.

In your body

Here are some common examples of prefixes in body-related words. You can see a nice mix of amounts, directions, and changes in these prefixes:

- ✔ **Ame**norrhea: Without period or menses, as in pregnancy
- ✔ **An**ovulatory: Ovaries not ovulating; can be hormonally induced
- ✔ **Bi**lateral: Lateral meaning side; both sides
- ✔ **Brady**cardia: Slow heart rate
- ✔ **Brady**arrhythmia: Slow irregular heartbeat
- ✔ **Circum**ferential: Around the outside
- ✔ **Dys**functional: Difficult or painful menstruation; dysfunctional uterine bleeding

- ✔ **Exo**cervix: Part of the cervix away from the uterus

- ✔ **Endo**cervix: Inner part of cervix, within the uterus

- ✔ **Hyper**tension: Excessive or high blood pressure

- ✔ **Hyper**emesis: Excessive vomiting

- ✔ **Hypo**tensive: Low or below normal blood pressure

- ✔ **Infra**umbilical: Below or beneath the umbilicus

- ✔ **Multi**loculated: A tumor or cyst having many or multiple locules, small spaces or cavities often filled with fluid

- ✔ **Olig**uria: Scanty, inadequate amount of urine production

- ✔ **Oligo**menorrhea: Scanty menstrual flow

- ✔ **Para**ovarian: Beside an ovary

- ✔ **peri**cardial: Around the heart

- ✔ **Peri**urethral: Around the opening of the urethra

- ✔ **Poly**dipsia: Excessive thirst (symptom of diabetes)

- ✔ **Poly**uria: Excessive urination (also symptom of diabetes)

- ✔ **Pseudo**cyst: A structure resembling a cyst; but not an actual cyst

- ✔ **Sub**costal: Beneath or under the ribs

- ✔ **Sub**umbilical: Area beneath or under the umbilicus

In the doctor's office and hospital

Check out this sampling of words you might hear around the physician's office or in the hospital ER:

- ✔ **Ab**duction: Moving a body part away from the point of origin

    This term is used in orthopedics to test range of motion of an arm or leg. In medical transcription, it is often dictated as "A-B-duction" to distinguish from "A-D-duction," meaning the opposite.

- ✔ **Ad**duction: Moving towards the point of origin; opposite of abduction; usually dictated or pronounced "A-D-duction."

- ✔ **Auto**logous bone graft: Bone taken from donor site on body to use as a graft on another part of the body

- ✔ **Dis**section: To cut or slice into two parts

- ✔ **Intra**uterine device: Contraceptive device inside or within uterus

- **Intra**venous: Within a vein; injection within a vein (not between)
- **Intra**muscular: Injection into a muscle, not between
- **Macro**scopic: Large enough to be seen with the naked eye
- **Multi**parous: Condition of having had many children
- **Peri**operative: Period of time around or during an operative procedure
- **Post**natal: After or following giving birth
- **Post**operative: Period of time following an operative procedure
- **Pre**operative: Period of time before an operative procedure
- **Pre**natal: Period of time before giving birth
- **Pre**menstrual: Period of time before a menstrual period begins
- **Pseudo**pregnancy: A false pregnancy
- **Tachy**cardia: Rapid or fast heart rate
- **Tachy**arrhythmia: Rapid or fast heart arrhythmia

In the pharmacy and research lab

Heaven knows there are tons of long, hard-to-spell, 25-cent words used in the pharmacy and the lab. Here's a quick taste:

- **Anti**-inflammatory: Agent opposing or fighting against inflammation
- **Contra**indication: Inadvisable, to be avoided

   In drug therapy, one drug might be contraindicated to another because of the effects of the use of both together.
- **Micro**scopic: Very small; only seen using a microscope
- **Neo**plasia: Condition of new or recent (cell) growth
- **Neo**plasm: New or recent growth; could be a tumor or cyst

Retro Root Rewind A–M

So you know the prefixes. Great! Now, can you remember the wide range of root words they match up with to create medical terms? Table 6-1 gives you a quick refresher course on roots from A–M. For the N–Z root words, see the end of Chapter 7.

Table 6-1	Recapping Root Words (A–M)
Root Word	**What It Means**
Abdomin/o	Abdomen
Aden/o	Gland
Adren/o	Adrenal gland
Alveoli/o	Air sac
Angi/o	Vessel
Arteri/o	Artery
Arteriol/o	Arteriole
Ather/o	Fatty degeneration
Arthr/o	Joint
Atri/o	Atrium
Audi/o	Hearing
Balan/o	Glans penis
Bio-	Life
Bronch/i, bronch/o	Bronchus
Bronchiol/o	Bronchiole
Carcin/o	Cancer
Cardi/o	Heart
Cellul/o	Cell
Cerebell/o	Cerebellum
Cerebr/i, cerebr/o	Cerebrum
Chol/e	Bile
Cholecyst/o	Gallbladder
Choledoch/o	Common bile duct
Chondr/i, chondr/o	Cartilage
Chrom/o	Color
Col/o	Colon
Colp/o	Vagina
Cost/o	Rib
Cry/o	Cold
Crypt/o	Hidden
Cutane/o	Skin
Cyan/o	Blue

Root Word	What It Means
Cysti, cyst/o	Bladder or cyst
Cyt/o	Cell
Dipl/o	Double, twice
Duoden/o	Duodenum
Encephal/o	Brain
Enter/o	Intestine
Episi/o	Vulva
Esophag/o	Esophagus
Erythr/o	Red
Fibr/o	Fibers
Galact/o	Milk
Gastr/o	Stomach
Glyc/o	Sugar
Gynec/o	Female
Hemat/o	Blood
Hepat/o, hepatic/o	Liver
Heter/o	Other, different
Hidr/o	Sweat
Hist/o, histi/o	Tissue
Hom/o, home/o	Same, alike
Hydr/o	Water, wet
Hyster/o	Uterus
Iatr/o	Treatment
Ile/o	Ileum (intestine)
Ili/o	Ilium (pelvic bone)
Intestin/o	Intestine
Jejun/o	Jejunum
Kerat/o	Cornea of eye, horny tissue
Lacrima	Tears
Laryng/o	Larynx
Leuk/o	White
Lith/o	Stone or calculus
Lipid/o	Fat

(continued)

Table 6-1 *(continued)*

Root Word	What It Means
Lymph/o	Lymph vessels
Melan/o	Black
Mening/o	Meninges
Men/o	Menses, menstruation
Metr/a, metr/o	Uterus
Myel/o	Bone marrow or spinal cord
My/o	Muscle
Myring/o	Eardrum

Chapter 7

So It Shall Be in the End: Suffixes

*T*he suffix has a job that's as important as the prefix's and the root word's. It is a third clue to the mystery of each medical term. The suffix is always at the end of a word and usually indicates a procedure, a condition, or a disease. All medical terms have suffixes. The suffix is all business and tells us what is happening with a specific body part or system — usually what is wrong with the body or which procedure is being used to diagnose or fix it.

Common Suffixes

The scope of suffix meanings is extremely wide. Like prefixes, many suffixes have similar meanings to those used in plain old, everyday English, whereas some are wildly different. You will get to know the usual suspects of suffixes fairly quickly — the following three in particular.

-itis

The suffix *-itis* simply indicates an inflammation of some kind. The *-itis* is quite popular in medical terminology because it can be applied to just about any body part within any body system. Here's a quick sample:

✔ **Tonsillitis:** Inflammation of the tonsils

✔ **Bronchitis:** Inflammation of the bronchus

✔ **Arthritis:** Inflammation of a joint

-oma

Remember the goofy yet memorable David Letterman joke, "Oprah, Uma. Uma, Oprah."? Well, meet *-oma*. The *-oma* suffix can often stand for something certainly not as pretty as Uma Thurman: a tumor. It can also pertain to a neoplasm, or new growth. Again, *-oma* is one of the most versatile suffixes because a tumor or neoplasm can happen on or near any body part, in any body system. Some *-oma*s you might have heard of:

- **Carcinoma:** Malignant (cancerous) tumor or growth
- **Leiomyoma:** Benign (non-cancerous) tumor derived from smooth muscle. Commonly called a fibroid or fibroid tumor.
- **Melanoma:** Tumor of the *melanocytic* (melanocytes in the skin) system of the skin, a highly malignant and quickly metastasizing (spreading) tumor.

A tumor can be benign or malignant depending on the type and composition, and amount of cell division and growth.

-pathy

The last of the big three is the *-pathy* suffix, which indicates a disease process. Once again, the wide-ranging use of this suffix is made possible by the large number of body systems it can help describe.

- **Cardiomyopathy:** Disease process involving the muscles of the heart
- **Cardiopathy:** Disease process involving the heart
- **Neuropathy:** Disease process involving the nervous system
- **Osteopathy:** Disease process involving bone

And lots more suffixes

There are, of course, many, many more suffixes that are just as important as the big three, though they may not be quite as recognizable to you (yet). As with English terms, many of the suffixes make their terms into adjectives. Table 7-1 lists several you should get to know.

Table 7-1	Suffixes: Wrapping It Up
Suffix	*What It Means*
-ac, -ic, -al, -ous, -tic	Related to or pertaining to
-algia, -dynia	Pain, discomfort
-ate, -ize	Subject to, use
-cele	Protrusion (hernia)
-centesis	Surgical puncture to withdraw or aspirate fluid
-cle, -cule, -ule, -ulus	Small
-cyte	Cell
-desis	Surgical fusion or binding
-dynia	Pain
-ectomy	Cutting out, surgical removal
-emesis	Vomit
-emia	Pertaining to blood, a blood condition
-ent, -er, -ist	Person, agent
-esis, -ia, -iasis, -ity, -osis, -sis, -tion, -y	State of or condition of
-form, -oid	Looking like, resembling, or shaped like
-genesis	A beginning process, origin of
-genic	Produced by
-gram	A written record
-graph	Instrument used to record
-graphy	Process of recording
-ism	Condition or theory
-lysis	Destruction, breakdown, or separation
-malacia	Softening
-megaly	Enlargement
-meter	Instrument used to measure
-metry	Process of measuring
-ologist	One who studies, a specialist
-ology	Study of, process of study
-opsy	To view
-otomy	Process of incision or cutting into

(continued)

Table 7-1 *(continued)*

Suffix	What It Means
-ostomy, -stomy	Artificial surgical opening
-penia	Lack of or deficiency
-pexy, -pexis	Surgical fixation
-phagia, -phagy	Eating
-phobia	Morbid fear of or intolerance
-plasia	Formation, development
-plasty	Surgical reconstruction, or shaping of
-plegia	Paralysis
-pnea	Breathing
-poiesis	Production or manufacture of
-ptosis	Downward displacement, or drooping
-rrhage, -rrhagia	Excessive flow or discharge
-rrhaphy	Suturing in place, fixation
-rrhea	Flow or discharge
-rrhexis	Rupture or breaking away
-sclerosis	Hardening
-scope	Instrument used to visually examine
-scopy	Process of visual examination
-spasm	Sudden or involuntary
-tome	Instrument
-tripsy	Crushing
-trophic, -trophy	Growth or development

The suffixes, *-rrhagia* or *rrhage*, *-rrhaphy*, *-rrhea*, and *-rrhexis* are known as The Four Rs. All four are difficult to pronounce and are almost always misspelled — usually with one *r* being left out.

Matching Suffixes to Situations

Tired yet? Hang in there just a bit longer, because now it's time to take a look at some examples of suffixes in the real medical world. Let's start with the place closest to you: your own body.

In your body

- Acro**phobia**: Fear of heights
- Ane**mia**: Low hemoglobin in blood
- Ap**nea**: Condition of not breathing
- Cardio**megaly**: Enlargement of the heart
- Claustro**phobia**: Fear of enclosed or small area
- Col**ostomy**: Artificial opening into the colon
- Dia**rrhea**: Frequent flow of watery or loose stools
- Dys**phagia**: Painful or difficult eating (or swallowing)
- Dys**pnea**: Difficult or painful breathing
- Erythr**ocytes**: Red blood cells
- Gastro**dynia**: Stomach pain or discomfort
- Hemi**plegia**: Paralysis of one side of body
- Hemo**rrhage**: Excessive flow of blood
- Hepato**megaly**: Enlargement of the liver
- Hepatospleno**megaly**: Enlargement of the liver and spleen
- Hyper**emesis**: Excessive vomiting
- Ile**ostomy**: Artificial opening into the ileum
- Leuk**emia**: Blood condition of white blood cells
- Leuko**cytes**: White blood cells
- Meno**rrhea**: Heavy menstrual period
- My**algia**: Muscle pain
- Nephr**osis**: Kidney condition
- Ortho**pnea**: Inability to breathe properly except in an upright position
- Osteo**penia**: Deficiency in bone mass
- Photo**phobia**: Visual intolerance of light
- Quadri**plegia**: Paralysis of all four quadrants of the body
- Spleno**megaly**: Enlargement of the spleen
- Trache**ostomy**: Artificial opening into the trachea; follows a tracheotomy

In the doctor's office and hospital

- Abdomino**plasty**: Plastic surgery on the abdomen
- Amnio**centesis**: Procedure to withdraw fluid from amniotic sac during pregnancy
- Appendec**tomy**: Surgical removal of appendix
- Broncho**scope**: Instrument used to perform a bronchoscopy
- Cardio**gram**: Hard copy record of cardiography
- Cardio**graph**: Machine used to perform a cardiography
- Cardio**graphy**: Process of recording activity of the heart
- Hernio**rrhaphy**: Surgical fixation or repair of a hernia
- Hysterec**tomy**: Surgical removal of uterus
- Laparo**scope**: Instrument used to perform a laparoscopy
- Lapar**otomy**: Cutting into the abdomen
- Mammo**graphy**: Process of examination of breast tissue
- Myo**rrhaphy**: Suture or fixation of a muscle
- Myo**rrhexis**: Suturing of a ruptured muscle
- Naso**plasty**: Repair of deviated nasal septum
- Oste**otomy**: Cutting into bone
- Psych**ologist**: Person who studies psychology
- Rhino**plasty**: Nose job
- Trache**otomy**: Cutting into the trachea
- Urethro**pexy**: Surgical fixation of the urethra

Retro Root Rewind N–Z

If you read Chapter 6, you may remember that we left you hanging in the middle of the alphabet in our root word recap. Here is your chance to finish recalling all those righteous root words that match up to the myriad of prefixes and suffixes. Table 7-2 covers N–Z. For A–M, go back one chapter.

Table 7-2	Recapping Root Words (N–Z)
Root Word	**What It Means**
Nat/o	Birth
Necr/o	Death
Nephr/o	Kidney
Neur/o	Nerve
Oophor/o	Ovary
Orchid/o, orchi/o	Testis
Oss/eo, oss/i, ost/e, ost/eo	Bone
Path/o	Disease
Palat/o	Roof of mouth
Peritone/o	Peritoneum (membrane lining abdominal and pelvic cavities)
Pharmac/o	Drug
Pharyng/o	Pharynx (throat)
Phleb/o	Vein
Phren/o	Diaphragm
Pleur/o	Pleura, rib (side)
Pneum/a/o, pneum/ono, pneum/ato	Lungs
Poli/o	Gray matter of nervous system
Proct/o	Rectum, anus
Pulmon/o	Lungs
Pyel/o	Pelvis of kidney
Py/o	Pus
Rect/o	Rectum
Ren/i, ren/o	Kidney
Sacr/o	Sacrum
Salping/o	Fallopian tube
Sarc/o	Flesh
Scapul/o	Scapula
Sept/o	Infection
Splen/o	Spleen
Spondyl/o	Vertebra

(continued)

Table 7-2 *(continued)*

Root Word	What It Means
Stern/o	Sternum
Tend/o, ten/o	Tendon
Testicul/o	Testis
Therm/o	Heat
Thorac/o	Chest
Thym/o	Thymus
Thyr/o, thyroid/o	Thyroid gland
Tonsill/o	Tonsils
Trache/o	Trachea
Tympan/o	Eardrum
Ur/e, ur/ea, ur/eo, urin/o, ur/o	Urine
Urethr/o	Urethra
Ureter/o	Ureter
Vas/o	Vas deferens (tube that carries sperm from the epididymis to the urethra)
Vas/o, ven/o	Vein
Vesic/o	Bladder
Viscer/o	Viscera (internal organs)
Xanth/o	Yellow
Xer/o	Dry

Chapter 8

Hey, I Know You: Word Recognition

*G*etting the hang of medical prefixes, roots, and suffixes is just the beginning of reaching your goal of becoming a terminology expert. Once you do that, you can move on to general word recognition.

Root words remain the basic component of word building, and you can look directly to them to recognize all sorts of words that associate with specific body parts and regions. Because you have spent so much time going over these individual building blocks, you can now begin to use what you know to piece together the larger puzzle of knowing whole words.

All your memorization should be starting to pay off. By now, many medical words parts should be second nature to you, and you can use them to create all sorts of related words.

Before you jump headfirst into your medical dictionary, though, take a brief moment to give props to your Greek and Latin granddaddies for making it all possible. Although the wonders of modern medicine and language evolution have changed many terms to make them more applicable and comprehensive, remember that most medical terms *are* derivatives of Latin and Greek.

Blame it on Aristotle and Hippocrates. Approximately 75 percent of all medical terms are based on Latin or Greek terms.

Going back to Chapter 2 to the topic of etymology, you might recall (hopefully!) that all words have an origin and a history. A large portion of medical terms have Greek roots. Take a fairly common term, *hemorrhage*, as an example.

You might hear that word, but did you know you can thank the Greeks for it? *Hemorrhage* is a word with Greek origin indicating a rapid, uncontrollable loss of blood.

Imagine a quick look from head to toe of the human body. If you could magically turn your eyes into a full body scan machine, you would see that your body is divided into several regions and cavities. Hundreds of words are associated with each of these different locations and the body parts contained in them. Before you get started on the words associated with them, take a quick tour of the body regions.

First, envision the cranial cavity in the head, together with the brain. That round ball that is your head is probably already full of all sorts of words and terms (and hopefully many more after you've finished this book). The *thoracic* or chest cavity houses the lungs, heart, aorta, trachea, and esophagus. Next is the *abdominal* cavity containing the stomach, intestines, spleen, liver, pancreas, gallbladder, ureters, and kidneys. The *pelvic* cavity contains the bladder, urethra, uterus, ovaries, and vagina in the female (testes in the male), as well as part of the large intestine, and the rectum (in both). In the middle of the whole mix is the *spinal* cavity, which consists of the spinal column connected to the cranial cavity.

The Inside Story: Terms for Your Interior

Inside all these cavities, of course, lies a bounty of body part-related medical terms. All the root words and combining forms from Chapter 3 (and Chapters 6 and 7) can morph into all kinds of different words that explain everything from everyday common conditions and procedures to pathology and pharmacology.

Remember that you can take any root word or combining form and create several different medical terms.

Table 8-1 lists many examples of where these root words can take you on your medical terminology journey.

Table 8-1	Interior Affairs	
Root Word	*What It Means*	*Example(s)*
Abdomin/o	Abdomen	Abdominoplasty: Surgical repair or reconstruction of the abdomen

Angi/o	Vessel	Angioplasty: Surgical repair or reconstruction of a vessel
Arteri/o	Artery	Arterioplasty: Surgical repair or reconstruction of an artery
Arthr/o	Joint	Arthritis: Inflammation of a joint
		Arthroplasty: Surgical repair or reconstruction of a joint
Audi/o	Hearing	Audiometry: Measurement of hearing using an audiometer
Bio	Life	Biology: The study of life and living organisms
Bronch/i, bronch/o	Bronchus/lung	Bronchitis: Inflammation of the bronchus
		Bronchoscopy: Visual examination of the bronchus
Cardi/o	Heart	Cardiomegaly: Enlargement of the heart
		Cardiac: Pertaining to the heart
		Carditis: Inflammation of the heart
Cholecyst/o	Gallbladder	Cholecystectomy: Removal of the gallbladder
		Cholecystitis: Inflammation of the gallbladder
Chondr/i, chondr/o	Cartilage	Chondromalacia: Softening of cartilage
Col/o	Colon	Colonoscopy: Visual examination of the colon
		Colonoscope: Instrument used in colonoscopy
Cry/o	Cold	Cryobiology: Branch of biology dealing with effects of low temperatures
Cysti, cyst/o	Bladder, or cyst	Cystectomy: Surgical removal of a simple cyst or of the urinary bladder
		Cystitis: Inflammation of the bladder
		Cystogram: Radiograph of the bladder
		Cystopexy: Surgical fixation of the bladder to abdominal wall

(continued)

Table 8-1 *(continued)*

Root Word	What It Means	Example(s)
Cyt/o	Cell	Cytology: Study of cells
Duoden/o	Duodenum (first section of small intestine)	Duodenotomy: Surgical cutting into the duodenum
		Duodenectomy: Surgical removal of the duodenum
		Duodenitis: Inflammation of the duodenum
Encephal/o	Brain	Encephalitis: Inflammation of the brain
Episi/o	Vulva	Episiotomy: Surgical cutting of the vulva
Esophag/o	Esophagus	Esophagitis: Inflammation of the esophagus
		Esophagogastroduodenoscopy (EGD): Visual examination of the esophagus, stomach, and duodenum by scope
Erythr/o	Red	Erythrocytes: Red blood cells
		Erythema: Reddening of the skin
Galact/o	Milk	Galactorrhea: Spontaneous flow of milk when nursing
Gastr/o	Stomach	Gastritis: Inflammation of the stomach
		Gastrectomy: Surgical removal of the stomach
		Gastrodynia: Stomach ache
Glyc/o	Sugar	Glycosuria: Sugar in the urine
Gynec/o	Female	Gynecologist: Physician who studies and treats diseases of female reproductive organs
Hemat/o	Blood	Hematocyte: Blood cell
Hepat/o, hepatic/o	Liver	Hepatitis: Inflammation of the liver
Heter/o	Other, different	Heterosexual: Sexually attracted to the opposite sex
Hist/o, histi/o	Tissue	Histology: Study and function of tissue

Root Word	What It Means	Example(s)
Hom/o, home/o	Same, alike	Homosexual: Sexually attracted to the same sex
Hydr/o	Water, wet	Hydromassage: Massage by means of moving water
Hyster/o	Uterus	Hysterectomy: Surgical removal of the uterus
Ile/o	Ileum (intestine)	Ileostomy: Artificial opening into the ileum
		Ileitis: Inflammation of the ileum
ili/o	Ilium (pelvic bone)	Ilioinguinal: Pertaining to the ilium and inguinal regions
Jejun/o	Jejunum (in small intestine)	Jejunitis: Inflammation of the jejunum
		Jejunostomy: Artificial opening into the jejunum
Lacrima	Tears	Lacrimatory: Causing a flow of tears
Laryng/o	Larynx	Laryngitis: Inflammation of the larynx
		Laryngectomy: Surgical removal of the larynx
Leuk/o	White	Leukocyte: White blood cell
Lith/o	Stone or calculus	Lithotripsy: Crushing of a stone or calculus
Men/o	Menstruation	Menorrhea: Menstrual flow
		Menorrhagia: Excessive or heavy menstrual flow
Myel/o	Bone marrow or spinal cord	Myelogram: Recording of the spinal cord
My/o	Muscle	Myositis: Inflammation of a muscle
		Myalgia: Pain in a muscle or painful muscle
Nat/o	Birth	Prenatal: Before birth
		Postnatal: After birth
Necr/o	Death	Necrosis: Death of a cell
		Necrophobia: Morbid fear of death or dead bodies
Nephr/o	Kidney	Nephrectomy: Surgical removal of a kidney

(continued)

Table 8-1 *(continued)*

Root Word	What It Means	Example(s)
Neur/o	Nerve	Neurologist: Physician who studies and treats conditions of the nervous system
Oophor/o	Ovary	Oophorectomy: Surgical removal of an ovary
		Oophoritis: Inflammation of an ovary
Orchid/o, orchi/o	Testis	Orchialgia: A pain in the testicle
		Orchiectomy: Surgical removal of a testicle
Peritone/o	Peritoneum	Peritoneal: Pertaining to the peritoneum
		Peritonitis: Inflammation of the peritoneum
Pharyng/o	Pharynx	Pharyngitis: Inflammation of the pharynx (sore throat)
Pleur/o	Pleura, rib (side)	Pleurisy: Inflammation of the lining of the chest cavity
		Pleurolysis: Surgical separation of pleural adhesions
Pneum/a/o/ato/ono	Lungs	Pneumonitis: Inflammation of the lung
Proct/o	Rectum, anus	Proctologist: Physician who studies and treats diseases of rectum and anus
Pulmon/o	Lungs	Pulmonary: Pertaining to the lungs
Pyel/o	Renal pelvis	Pyelography: Radiograph (x-ray) of the pelvis of the kidney
		Pyelolithotomy: Removal of a stone from the kidney pelvis
Rect/o	Rectum	Rectosigmoid: Pertaining to the rectum and sigmoid
Salping/o	Fallopian tube	Salpingectomy: Surgical removal of a fallopian tube
Sarc/o	Flesh	Sarcoid: Resembling flesh

Root Word	What It Means	Example(s)
Splen/o	Spleen	Splenomegaly: Enlargement of the spleen
		Splenectomy: Surgical removal of the spleen
Tend/o, ten/o	Tendon	Tendinitis (or tendonitis): Inflammation of a tendon
Testicul/o	Testis	Testicular: Pertaining to a testis or testicle
		Testitis: Inflammation of a testis
Thorac/o	Chest	Thoracotomy: Incision into the chest cavity
		Thoracentesis: Surgical puncture into chest cavity
Tonsill/o	Tonsils	Tonsillectomy: Surgical removal of tonsils
		Tonsillitis: Inflammation of the tonsils
Ureter/o	Ureter	Ureterolithotomy: Removal of a calculus (stone) from a ureter by means of incision
		Ureteropelvic: Pertaining to the ureter and pelvis of the kidney
Urethr/o	Urethra	Urethritis: Inflammation of the urethra
		Urethropexy: Surgical fixation of the urethra
Vas/o	Vas deferens	Vasectomy: Surgical removal of portion of vas deferens for male sterilization
Viscer/o	Viscera (organs)	Viscerography: Radiography of the viscera

Terms for the Outside of Your Body

Whew! Now let's take a look at some of the words you can conjure for the exterior of your body. Table 8-2 is your ticket.

Table 8-2	Out of Bounds: External Terminology	
Root Word	*What It Means*	*Example(s)*
Blephar/o	Eyelid or eyelash	Blepharoplasty: Surgical repair of the eyelids
Cephal/o	Head	Cephalocentesis: Surgical puncture of the head (skull)
		Cephalomegaly: Enlargement of the head (skull)
Cervic/o	Neck or cervix	Cervicodynia: Pain in the neck
		Cervicitis: Inflammation of the cervix
Cheil/o, chil/o	Lip	Cheilophagia: Biting of the lips
Derm/a/o, dermat/o	Skin	Dermatitis: Inflammation of the skin
		Dermatologist: Physician who studies and treats diseases of the skin
		Dermatome: Instrument used for cutting thin skin slices for skin grafting
Dors/i, dors/o	Back or posterior	Dorsalgia: Pain in the back
Gingiv/o	Gums in mouth	Gingivitis: Inflammation of the gums
Inguin/o	Groin	Inguinodynia: Pain in the groin
Irid/o	Iris of eye	Iridectomy: Surgical removal of the iris
Lapar/o	Abdomen, loin, flank	Laparotomy: Cutting into the abdomen
		Laparoscopy: Visual examination into the abdomen
Lingu/o	Tongue	Sublingual: Under the tongue
Mamm/a, mamm/o	Breast	Mammoplasty: Surgical repair or reconstruction of the breast
Mast/o	Breast	Mastectomy: Surgical removal of the breast
Odont/o	Teeth	Odontalgia: Toothache
Onych/o	Nails	Onychophagia: Habit of biting the nails
		Onychomalacia: Softening of the nails
Ophthalm/o, ocul/o	Eyes	Ophthalmologist: Physician studying eyes and treatment of eye disease
Optic/o, opt/o	Seeing, sight	Optician: One who fills the ophthalmologist's prescription for corrective eye glasses

Root Word	What It Means	Example(s)
Or/o	Mouth	Orolingual: Pertaining to the mouth and tongue
Ot/o	Ear	Otitis media: Inflammation of the middle ear
		Otodynia: Earache
Pelv/o	Pelvis	Pelvimetry: Measurement of dimensions and capacity of the pelvis
Pod/o	Foot	Podarthritis: Inflammation of the joints of the foot
Rhin/o	Nose	Rhinoplasty: Nose job
		Rhinorrhea: Discharge of mucus from the nose (runny nose)
Stomat/o	Mouth	Stomatitis: Inflammation of the oral mucosa or lining of the mouth
Thorac/o	Chest	Thoracentesis: Surgical puncture into the chest cavity
		Thoracotomy: Surgical incision into the chest cavity

Table 8-3		Quick Glance: Pathology
Root Word	What It Means	Example(s)
Aden/o	Gland	Adenomegaly: Enlargement of a gland
		Adenitis: Inflammation of a gland
Atri/o	Atrium	Atriomegaly: Abnormal enlargement of an atrium of the heart
Carcin/o	Cancer	Carcinogen: A cancer-producing substance
Cheir/o, chir/o	Hand	Cheiromegaly: Abnormal enlargement (megaly) of the hand
Cholecyst/o	Gallbladder	Cholelithiasis: Stones in the gallbladder
Choledoch/o	Common bile duct	Choledocholithiasis: Stones in the common bile duct of the gallbladder
Cyan/o	Blue	Cyanosis: Bluish discoloration of the skin
		Cyanotic: Pertaining to or characterized by cyanosis

(continued)

Table 8-3 *(continued)*

Root Word	What It Means	Example(s)
Cysti, cyst/o	Bladder or cyst	Cystocele: Hernial protrusion of urinary bladder through vaginal wall
Dipl/o	Double, twice	Diplopia: The condition of double vision
Encephal/o	Brain	Encephalopathy: A disorder or disease of the brain
Hemat/o	Blood	Hematemesis: Vomiting of blood
Hepat/o, hepatic/o	Liver	Hepatomegaly: Enlargement of the liver
Hydr/o	Water, wet	Hydropenia: Deficiency of water in the body (dehydration)
Melan/o	Black	Melanoma: Black-colored tumor or growth
Necr/o	Death	Necrosis: Condition of death of a cell
Nephr/o	Kidney	Nephrolithiasis: Condition of kidney stones
Path/o	Disease	Pathology: Branch of medicine that deals with the study of disease and its effects
		Pathologist: Physician who diagnoses diseases by examining tissues and cells under a microscope. Also performs autopsies.
Pneum/ato, pneum/ono	Lungs	Pneumoconiosis: Condition of abnormal deposits of dusts or other matter in the lungs
Salping/o	Fallopian tube	Hydrosalpinx: Accumulation of fluid in a fallopian tube
Sept/o	Infection	Septicemia: Toxins or pathogenic organisms in the blood (blood poisoning)
Ureter/o	Ureter	Ureterolith: Calculus or stone lodged in the ureter
Urethr/o	Urethra	Urethrorrhea: Abnormal discharge from the urethra
Viscer/o	Viscera (organs)	Visceromegaly: Enlargement of internal organs, also called organomegaly

Chapter 9

Deconstruction Junction: Breaking Down Words

A necessary and important component to learning medical terminology and medical terms is being able to break down or dissect a word to establish its meaning. Knowing your word parts and how to break down a medical term by its word parts is a vital method you can use to understand its definition. This means hard-to-pronounce or long medical terms used by physicians and healthcare workers are *not* as difficult as they seem.

When you understand a word part and understand the word part's meaning, it is easy to analyze the definition of a medical term. Many medical words are very close in spelling but have different meanings. When you know the correct meaning of a word, there is less chance of using a sound-alike word inappropriately.

When in doubt, look it up in a medical dictionary.

Now, let's take on some larger words and try to break them down using the rules.

Finding Parts of Words

Don't worry — you're not backtracking, you're just reminding yourself about the three major parts of every medical term so that you can more easily discover its meaning.

Identifying word elements

At the beginning of a medical term you often (but not always) find the prefix, which can indicate the direction, the where, the when and the amount.

Next comes the root word, indicating the body part involved. Some root word meanings are obvious and easy to understand, like *arteri/o* for artery, *abdomin/o* for abdomen, *testicul/o* for testicle, and *tonsill/o* for tonsil. Many are not so easy: What about *blephar/o* for eyelids, *aden/o* for gland, *nephr/o* for kidney, *hepat/o* for liver, or *oophor/o* for ovary? Obviously, you're going to have to break out your best memorization skills for words like these.

The suffix at the end of a term is often your first clue to the definition of the term. It can indicate a procedure, a condition, or a disease.

There is *always* a suffix at the end of a medical term.

The meaning of a suffix, just as with some root words, may not be obvious. It's important to remember that the suffix always has the same meaning, no matter what root word it's tacked on to.

The suffix, then, is the first place to look when trying to analyze or break down a medical term. From the suffix, back up to the prefix, if there is one, and finally, look at the root word.

Defining the prefix

The prefix and suffix are "adjectives," in a way, telling you something about the root word in the middle. Changing the prefix or the suffix changes the meaning of the term.

Let's look at some commonly used prefixes, *pre-* (before), *peri-* (during), and *post-* (after or following), all coupled with the same term. Watch how the prefix changes the time frame. We can use the word *operative* for example, beginning with *preoperative*, referring to the time period or events before an operative procedure. Changing the prefix to *peri-* would be *perioperative*, indicating the time or the events around or during an operation. Then changing the prefix to *post-* would result in *postoperative*, meaning the time or events after the surgery is completed. By using the three different prefixes, each of these words sound somewhat alike but are quite different in their meaning.

Some prefixes often mistaken one for another are the prefixes *ab-*, meaning "away from" and *ad-*, meaning "towards" or "in the direction of."

Remember *abduction*, a kidnapping, or being taken away, as a memory key to tell the two apart.

Another example is the prefix *dys-*, often used in medical terms. Think of *dysfunctional* (not the *dis* in *discomfort*). *Dys-* used as a prefix in front of a medical term means "difficult," "bad," or "painful."

The prefix *inter-*, meaning "between or among," is often mistaken for *intra-*, which means "within or inside." Think of an *interstate* highway, winding between and among states. For *intra-*, think of an *intrauterine contraceptive device*, used within or inside the uterus.

The definition of a prefix is always the same, no matter what it's paired with.

Each time you see *intra-* before a root word, it always means "within or inside of." *Inter-* always means "between or among."

Prefixes are joined to a root word without the use of a hyphen, even when a double vowel results as in *perioperative, intrauterine*. The only exception to this rule is that a hyphen is used when the prefix joins up with a proper name: *non-Hodgkin's lymphoma*.

Defining the root word

The root word describes the body parts involved in the medical term. Take a look at some common examples.

- ✔ **Arthro:** Joint
- ✔ **Myelo:** Bone marrow
- ✔ **Myo:** Muscle
- ✔ **Neuro:** Nerve
- ✔ **Osteo:** Bone

As always, a little memory work is needed here.

Medical terms always have a suffix *but not always a prefix*. Some medical terms have a combination of two or more root words, coupling multiple body parts together: *hepatospleno* comes from *hepato* (liver) and *spleno* (spleen).

Identifying the combining vowel

The *combining vowel*, usually an *o*, joins the root word to a suffix. If a suffix begins with a vowel, the combining vowel *o* is not used, because it would create a double vowel.

Take the root word *neuro* (for "nerve," right?) as an example. Let's join it to the suffix *-itis*, which means "inflammation." Using the combining vowel *o* to join these together, we would have *neuroitis*, which is not only difficult to pronounce but also contains a double vowel. Therefore, the *o* is dropped, and inflammation of a nerve becomes *neuritis*.

Defining the suffix

As you know, the suffix indicates a procedure, disease, disorder, or condition, and you look at it first. For example, the suffix *-itis* is common. It means "inflammation," so every time you see *-itis*, you know it means something is inflamed. Taking a word that we know — tonsil — we know that *tonsillitis* means "inflammation of the tonsil." *Gastr/o* is the root word for "stomach," so *gastritis* is "inflammation of the stomach."

The commonly used suffix *-ectomy* means "surgical removal or excision of." When you put *-ectomy* with *tonsil*, you have *tonsillectomy*, removal of the tonsils. *Gastrectomy* would therefore be what? Right: Surgical removal of the stomach (yikes).

The word tonsil (or tonsils) has only one *l*, but when we make it into a combining form such as *tonsillitis* or *tonsillectomy*, the *l* is doubled. *Tonsillitis* is a commonly misspelled medical word. More memory work!

Suffixes as "adjectives" help describe the root word. For instance, the suffixes *-al, -ic, -ous,* and *-eal* are all suffixes that mean "pertaining to." The suffix *-ologist* refers to "one who studies or practices a specialized medical field." The suffix *-ology* is "the study of." The common suffix *-pathy* means "disease."

Take an easily identifiable root word, *cardio* or *cardiac,* meaning "heart," and apply different suffixes. *Cardiology* is the study of heart diseases. The *cardiologist* is the physician who practices cardiology, and *cardiopathy* means some form of heart disease. *Neurology,* then, is the study of nerves or the nervous system, and the *neurologist* is the physician who specializes in neurology. Any disease of the nervous system or the nerves is *neuropathy*.

Going Deeper into Suffixes

Check out some more suffix examples. Suffixes related to procedures include -*centesis*, referring to surgical puncture to remove fluid for diagnostic purposes or to remove excess fluid. That means *abdominocentesis* is surgical puncture of the abdominal cavity.

The suffix -*ectomy* means "surgical removal of." When you see -*ectomy* at the end of any term, no matter how long or how difficult or confusing the first part of the word is, it means surgical removal of something. Another term we all know that end in -*ectomy* is *appendectomy*, surgical removal of the appendix.

But, sadly, it's not always that easy. Take a look at a more complicated word and then break it down. How about the word *salpingo-oophorectomy*? The -*ectomy* we know indicates the surgical removal of something. But what? *Salpingo* is the root word referring to the fallopian tube; *oophoro* is the root word for ovary. Therefore, *salpingo-oophorectomy* is surgical removal of a fallopian tube and ovary. Surgical removal of an ovary only would be *oophorectomy*.

The shrewd among you may have noticed this: There is a hyphen in salpingo-oophorectomy. This is there mainly to aid with pronunciation and to avoid a triple "o" vowel with the combining of the two roots. The word can also be expressed as *oophorosalpingectomy*, which means the same thing.

Another suffix related to procedures is -*graphy*, meaning the process of recording a picture or a record. *Radiography* is the process of recording a picture by radiograph or an X-ray. Suffixes -*gram* and -*graph* are used to describe the finished product, the recording or picture. An *arteriography* is the process of recording the picture of arteries. The *arteriogram* or *arteriograph* is the film that is produced by the arteriography.

The suffix -*ostomy* means to surgically create an artificial opening or *stoma*. A *colostomy* is a surgical creation of an opening between the colon and the body surface. The root word *colo* means colon. The suffix -*otomy* means "surgical cutting into," or a surgical incision. In order, then, to perform a *tracheostomy* (the surgical creation of an opening in the trachea), a *tracheotomy* (the surgical incision into the trachea) must be performed.

It is important to know the difference between "ostomy" and "otomy" — there is only one letter difference, but a big difference in the meaning.

The suffix *-plasty* means "surgical repair." The rule of thumb to remember here is when you hear or see *-plasty* think of the plastic surgeon, because, in most cases, *-plasty* surgical procedures *are* performed by the plastic surgeon. A term associated with this suffix is *mammoplasty*. The root word *mammo* refers to the breast. A *reduction mammoplasty* would be surgical reduction in the size of the breast. Another commonly used suffix with regards to procedures is *-scopy*. This involves the visual examination of the interior of a body cavity or organ using an endoscope. The *endoscope* is the instrument, and *endoscopy* is the actual visual examination being performed with the endoscope.

In medicine today, more and more diagnostic procedures are being performed using the endoscopic method. Endoscopic surgery is less invasive. Small portals are made into skin, and the laparoscope provides visualization for excisions to be made through these small portals — as opposed to a full thickness, muscle-splitting incision to fully open up (in most cases) the abdominal wall.

Female sterilizations, hysterectomies, gallbladder removal, and appendectomies, just to name a few, are now being done laparoscopically. Less time is spent in the hospital, and the recovery period is reduced by as much as a month. For example, a gallbladder removed by routine upper abdominal incision requires a recovery period of four to six weeks; done laparoscopically, with only portals to heal, the time is cut to two weeks.

Suffixes related to conditions are used over and over again. You have already covered a few, but let's look at some. We have *-algia*, meaning "pain and suffering." *Arthralgia* would refer to the pain and suffering of joints. *Myalgia* means "pain or suffering in the muscle." The suffix *-dynia* also means "pain." The word *gastrodynia* (*gastro* is a root word for "stomach") means "pain in the stomach."

We already know *-itis* means "inflammation." You can have *gastritis, tonsillitis, laryngitis, thyroiditis, neuritis, cellulitis, dermatitis, colitis, enteritis,* and *arthritis* (though you certainly wouldn't want to). You could have an *-itis* of almost any part of your body.

Inflammation has two *m*'s, but inflamed has one.

The suffix *-malacia* means "abnormal softening," most often used referring to bone disorders, but it does mean abnormal softening, and *arteriomalacia* refers to abnormal softening of the walls of an artery or arteries.

The suffix *-megaly* means "large" or "enlarged." It can be coupled with many body parts or organs. *Cardiomegaly* means enlargement of the heart, *splenomegaly* enlargement of a spleen. *Hepatomegaly* is enlargement of the liver. *Thyromegaly* would be enlargement of the thyroid gland. And *hepatosplenomegaly* would be enlargement of the liver *and* spleen, a double-barreled root word.

The suffix -*osis* means "a disease or abnormal condition," a general suffix associated with many of the root words. *Gastrosis* means a disease (any disease) of the stomach. *Scoliosis* is a curvature of the spine. *Diverticulosis* means outpouchings of the intestinal wall. *Psychosis* (*psyche* is the root word for "mind") covers many varieties of mental disorders.

Adding Up Individual Word Meanings

Just as in a math problem, you can add up the parts of a word and get one coherent answer, one complete meaning. Here's one example to get you started: Break the word *gastroenterologist* into root words and suffixes:

gastroenterologist = gastro + entero + logist

Look at the suffix first: -*logist* says this is a person, the physician. Now go back to the beginning. *Gastro* is the root word for stomach, and *entero* is the root word for intestines. Broken down, then, a gastroenterologist is a physician who studies and treats diseases of the stomach and intestines, performing a medical service known as *gastroenterology*.

With two root words, the meaning of both root words must be researched to know the true meaning of the term.

Let's take a trip through the body to find some not so easy terms. Using the rules of dissection, you should be able decipher some brainteasers.

- ✔ **Ana/tomy:** -tomy ("process of cutting") + ana ("apart") = study of body structure (to study, one must cut up or dissect)
- ✔ **Auto/opsy:** -opsy ("to view") + auto ("self") = examination of body after death (yes, it's a stretch)
- ✔ **Bio/logy:** -logy ("the study of") + bio ("life") = study of living things
- ✔ **Cerebro/malacia:** -malacia ("softening") + cerebro ("brain") = softening of the brain
- ✔ **Cerebro/vascul/ar:** -ar ("pertaining to") + cerebro ("brain") + vasculo ("vessel") = pertaining to the brain and blood vessels
- ✔ **Choledocho/litho/tripsy:** -tripsy ("crushing") + choledocho ("common bile duct of the gallbladder") + litho ("stone") = crushing of stones in the common bile duct of the gallbladder
- ✔ **Chondro/malacia:** -malacia ("softening") + chondro ("cartilage") = softening of cartilage
- ✔ **Chondr/oma: -oma** ("mass or tumor") + chondro ("cartilage") = tumor of cartilage

- **Costo/chondr/al:** -al ("pertaining to") + costo ("rib") + chondro ("cartilage") = pertaining to the ribs and cartilage

- **Crani/otomy:** -otomy ("cutting into") + cranio ("skull") = cutting into the skull

- **Dermat/itis:** -itis ("inflammation") + dermato ("skin") = inflammation of the skin

- **Dermato/plasty:** -plasty ("surgical reconstruction") + dermato ("skin") = surgical reconstruction of the skin

- **Encephalo/pathy:** -pathy ("disease") + encephalo ("brain") = brain disease

- **Glyc/emia:** -emia ("blood condition") + glyco ("sugar") = sugar in the blood

  Then, by adding prefixes to glycemia, we get

  Hyper/glyc/emia: -hyper ("excessive") = excessive sugar in blood

  Hypo/glyc/emia: -hypo ("insufficient") = insufficient or low amount of sugar in the blood

- **Hemi/gastr/ectomy:** -ectomy ("surgical removal of") + hemi ("half") + gastro ("stomach") = surgical removal of half the stomach

- **Hemo/lysis:** -lysis ("breakdown or distruction") + hemo ("blood") = breakdown of blood

- **Hemat/emesis:** -emesis ("vomiting") + hemato ("blood") = vomiting of blood

- **Hyper/cholesterol/emia:** -emia ("blood condition") + hyper ("excessive or above normal") + cholesterol = excessive amount of cholesterol in blood

- **Hyper/hidr/osis:** -osis ("abnormal condition") + hyper ("excessive or above normal") + hidro ("sweat") = excessive secretion of sweat or excessive sweating

- **Hystero/salpingo/gram:** -gram ("a record") + hystero ("uterus") + salpingo ("fallopian tube") = X-ray record of the uterus and fallopian tubes

- **Intra/cranial:** -cranial ("pertaining to the skull") + intra ("within") = pertaining to within the skull

- **Labio/glosso/pharyng/eal:** - eal ("pertaining to") + labio ("lips") + glosso ("tongue") + pharyngo ("pharynx") = pertaining to the lips, tongue, and throat

- **Laryngo/tracheo/bronch/itis:** -itis ("inflammation") + laryngo ("larynx") + trachea ("trachea") + broncho ("bronchus") = inflammation of the larynx, trachea, and bronchus (*croup*)

✔ **Leio/myo/sarcoma:** -sarcoma ("malignant tumor") + leio ("smooth") + myo ("muscle") = malignant tumor of smooth muscle

✔ **Neur/itis:** -itis ("inflammation") + neuro ("nerve") = inflammation of a nerve

✔ **Para/nasal:** -nasal ("pertaining to nose") + para ("beside or near") = beside or near the nose

✔ **Peri/neur/itis:** -itis ("inflammation") + peri ("around") + neuro ("nerve") = inflammation around a nerve

✔ **Post/mortem:** -mortem ("death") + post ("following or after") = after death

✔ **Presby/opia:** -opia ("vision") + presby ("old age") = vision impaired due to aging

✔ **Presbycusis:** -cusis ("hearing") + presby ("old age") = diminished hearing due to aging

✔ **Thrombo/phleb/itis:** -itis ("inflammation") + thrombo ("clot") + phlebo ("vein") = inflammation of a vein with clot formation

Chapter 10

An Org Chart to Live By: Organization of the Body

. . . .

In This Chapter

▶ Distinguishing the different branches of science that help you study the body

▶ Discovering the building blocks of the body

▶ Getting to know anatomical regions, planes, and cavities

. . . .

*B*efore we get into the real nitty-gritty of the source of all these magnificent medical terms — your body, that is — you may want to first get to know the big picture of your body. In this chapter, we review the structure and organization of the body. The body appears to be a solid structure from the outside. Inside, body regions, organs, and cavities fit nicely together to provide that solid structure.

Looking at the Big Picture

There are all sorts of ways to look at the human body. You can study it from different angles, both literally and figuratively. Let's start with the figurative, as in the different kinds of science used to analyze the body. Then later, you can move on the some more concrete ways of looking at your beautiful bod.

The branches of science that cover the study of the body are as follows:

✔ **Anatomy** means "cutting apart." This is the science that studies the structure of the body and the relationships of its parts to each other. The "cutting apart" is the method used (*dissection*) to study the structure of the human body.

✔ **Biology** is the study of all forms of life and living things.

✔ **Embryology** studies the origin (beginnings) and the development of an organism. This covers from the 2nd to the 8th week after conception, which is referred to as the *embryonic stage*. After eight weeks, the developing organism is known as a *fetus*.

 ✔ **Histology** studies the body microscopically — the minute structures and their composition, plus the functions of normal cells, tissue, and organs.

 ✔ **Pathology** studies the changes caused by disease to the structures of the body or changes due to disease that alter the functions of the body.

 ✔ **Physiology** studies the normal activity and functions of the body.

Cells

The *cell* is the basic, smallest unit of life. Cells that perform similar functions join together, or group together, to form *tissue*. Groups of different types of tissue join together to form an *organ*. Groups of organs that work together to perform a complex function, form a *body system*.

The body is maintained by metabolism (*meta* means "change," *bolus* refers to "mass," and *ism* is "a condition"). *Metabolism* consists of the total processes of *anabolism* (*ana* means to build up) and *catabolism* (*cata* means to break down). When metabolism stops, an organism dies.

Each of us has trillions of cells that vary in size and shape according to their purpose or function. Specialized cells are responsible for the functions of growth, secretions, excretions, nutrition, and reproduction. Mechanical, chemical, and nervous stimulation activate the cells. The shapes of most typical cells are as follows:

 ✔ **Epithelial or skin cell:** May be square and flat

 ✔ **Fat cell:** Contains large vacant spaces for fat storage

 ✔ **Muscle cell:** Long and slender

 ✔ **Nerve cell:** May be long and have fingerlike extensions, which carry impulses

Each cell has a *membrane*, forming the exterior boundary; *cytoplasm* that makes up the body of the cell; and a *nucleus*, the small control center of the cell that contains the *chromosomes*. There are 46 chromosomes (23 pairs) in a human cell. *Genes* are regions within the chromosomes. Each chromosome has thousands of genes that all determine hereditary characteristics. Each gene is composed of *DNA* (*deoxyribonucleic acid*), the chemical that regulates the activities of the cell. The mature *reproductive* (sex) cell has only 23 chromosomes, and at conception, the male and female sex cells join together to contribute to innumerable possible combinations. That's why no two individuals are alike, except for identical twins.

Tissues

In the building blocks of body structures, cells of similar characteristics and specific tasks join together to form tissue. The body is made up of four different types of tissue:

- ✔ **Connective tissue** supports and encases body structures. It is the most widespread kind of tissue throughout the body. It holds organs in place and connects body parts to each other. The main types of connective tissue include *bone* that supports the body; *cartilage*, firm but bendable; *dense fibrous* that makes up the tendons and ligaments; *loose* that connects adjoining structures; and *apidose* tissue that pads and protects, stores fat, and insulates the body against heat loss.

- ✔ **Epithelial tissue:** Found in the skin and in the lining of blood vessels, this makes up the outer covering of external and internal body surfaces (such as skin and mucous membranes) and the lining of the digestive, respiratory, and urinary tracts.

- ✔ **Muscle tissue** provides movement. The main function of muscle tissue is to contract.

- ✔ **Nerve tissue** conducts impulses to and from the brain and is composed of nerve cells called neurons. Nervous tissue needs more oxygen and more nutrients than any other body tissue.

Organs and Systems

When two or more kinds of tissue work together to perform a specific function, you have an organ. For example, the skin is an organ made up of connective, nerve, and epithelial tissue.

Although organs act as units, they do not function alone. Several organs join together to form a system and perform a body function. Each system has a special function.

Some of the major body systems include the following:

- ✔ **The cardiovascular system** includes the heart and blood vessels and carries the blood throughout the body.

- ✔ **The digestive or gastrointestinal system** includes the mouth, esophagus, stomach, and small and large intestines. This system digests and absorbs food and excretes waste.

- ✔ **The endocrine system** is made up of a variety of glands and manufactures and distributes hormones.

- ✔ **The integumentary system** includes the hair, skin, nails, and sweat and oil glands.

- ✔ **The lymphatic system** works with the cardiovascular system to protect the body against disease-causing organisms.

- ✔ **The musculoskeletal system**, composed of bones, muscles, tendons, and ligaments, provides the framework for the body, supports organs, and permits movement in the body.

- ✔ **The reproductive systems**, the uterus, ovaries, testes, and prostate, provide for reproduction.

- ✔ **The respiratory system** includes the trachea, lungs, and bronchi and provides the exchange of gases, absorbs oxygen, and expels carbon dioxide.

- ✔ **The sensory or special senses system**, made up of the eyes, ears, nose, and mouth, along with the nervous system composed of the brain and spinal cord, processes stimuli and allows the body to act and respond.

- ✔ **The urinary system** manufactures and excretes urine.

Cavities of the Body

The body is not as solid a structure as it appears on the outside. It has five body cavities. Each *cavity* contains organs that are organized (no pun intended) in a neat and orderly fashion.

The five body cavities include the following:

- ✔ **The abdominal cavity** contains the stomach, intestines, liver, spleen, gallbladder, pancreas, ureters, and kidneys.

- ✔ **The cranial cavity,** the cavity inside the skull, or the *cranium*, contains the brain.

- ✔ **The pelvic cavity** contains the urinary bladder, urethra, uterus and vagina in the female, part of the large intestine, and the rectum.

- ✔ **The spinal cavity** consists of the spinal column connecting to the cranial cavity.

- ✔ **The thoracic or chest cavity** contains the esophagus, trachea, lungs, heart, and aorta. This cavity can be divided into two smaller areas. The *pleural cavity* surrounds the lungs. (Each pleural cavity is lined with a membrane called *pleura*. *Visceral pleura* is closest to the lungs. *Parietal pleura* is closest to the outer wall of the cavity.) The *mediastinum* is the area between the lungs. It contains the heart, aorta, trachea, esophagus, and thymus gland.

The cranial and spinal cavities are *dorsal* body cavities, as they are located on the back part of the body. The thoracic, abdominal, and pelvic cavities are *ventral* body cavities, as they are on the front or belly-side of the body.

The thoracic and abdominal cavities are separated by a muscular partition called the diaphragm. The abdominal and pelvic cavities are not separated and, to really confuse you, together they are frequently referred to as the *abdominopelvic cavity*.

Table 10-1 lists some root words related to body structure and organization.

Table 10-1		Roots of Structures	
Root	**What It Means**	**Example Term**	**What It Means**
Cyt/o	Cell	Cytology	Study of cells
Epitheli/o	Epithelium	Epithelioma	Tumor of the skin
Fibr/o	Fibrous	Fibrosis	Condition of the fibrous tissue
Hist/o	Tissue	Histologist	Physician who studies tissue
Lip/o	Fat	Liposuction	Removal of fat cells by suction
Myo	Muscle	Myositis	Inflammation of a muscle
Neur/o	Nerve	Neuropathy	Condition of the nerve
Organ/o	Organ	Organomegaly	Enlargement of an organ
Viscer/o	Internal organs	Viscera	Internal organs

Table 10-2 lists some suffixes pertaining to body structure and organization.

Table 10-2		Structural Suffixes	
Suffix	**What It Means**	**Example Term**	**What It Means**
-cyte	Cell	Erythrocyte	Red blood cell
-gen	Agent that causes	Carcinogen	Agent causing cancer
-genic	Producing	Carcinogenic	Has cancer-causing properties
-ologist	One who studies/ practices	Cytologist	Physician who studies cells

(continued)

Table 10-2 *(continued)*

Suffix	What It Means	Example Term	What It Means
-oma	Tumor or swelling	Myoma	Tumor in the muscle
-osis	Abnormal condition	Cytosis	Abnormal condition of cells
-pathy	Disease	Neuropathy	A disease of the nerves
-plasm	Growth or formation	Neoplasm	A new growth
-sar- coma	Malignant tumor	Myosarcoma	Malignant muscle tumor

Directional Terms and Anatomical Planes

An *anatomical plane* is an imaginary flat plate or field. Imagine a slice view through the body and you're on the right track. Anatomic planes provide further division of the body, again to identify a specific location or area. Visualize dividing the body in half, top from bottom, and then right from left, and finally front from back.

- ✔ **The frontal or coronal plane** is a vertical plane dividing the body into *anterior* (front) and *posterior* (back) portions.

- ✔ **The midsagittal plane** is a horizontal plane that divides the body into right and left halves at the body's midpoint.

- ✔ **The sagittal plane** is a vertical plane that passes from front to back, dividing the body into right and left sides.

- ✔ **The transverse plane** is a horizontal (cross-section) plane, parallel to the ground and through the waistline, dividing the body into upper and lower halves.

The anatomical planes of the body are used in radiology when specific body location or direction is necessary.

When thinking about all of these terms, planes, and regions, think of the body as if it is standing, arms at each side, with palms facing forward and the feet side by side. Whether a patient is standing, or lying down face up, the directional terms are always applied in the same manner.

Directional terms are used to pinpoint or specifically locate an area on the body.

When referring to the front of the body, the terms *anterior* and *ventral* are used. When referring to the back of the body, it's *posterior* and *dorsal*. With the waistline of the anatomical position as a guideline, above the waistline is referred to as *cephalad* ("head" or "upward") or *superior* ("above"). Below the waistline is referred to as *caudal* ("tail" or "downward") or *inferior* ("below"). Superior and inferior are also used to describe body parts in relation to one another in general.

The sides of the body are referred to as *lateral*, and the middle referred to as *medial*. The term *distal* refers to "away from the point of origin" (think of distance). *Proximal* refers to "nearest the point of origin" (close proximity). Distal and proximal are two directional terms that seem to pose problems. View the torso of the body as the point of origin. Using the arm as an example, the proximal portion of the arm is where the arm joins to the shoulder. The distal, or away-from, portion of the arm, would be the hand. In the leg, the upper thigh would be the proximal portion of the leg, and the foot would be the distal portion of the leg.

Directional terms can be joined together to provide a combined form. *Ipsilateral* pertains to one side, whereas *mediolateral* is a directional term meaning pertaining to the middle and one side (such as right mediolateral pain). It is often used in medical exams and surgical procedures. Here's one use of mediolateral: A right mediolateral abdominal incision would be an incision beginning at the middle of the abdomen and going toward the right side. A similar term is *lateromedial*. A lateromedial incision would be the same as a mediolateral one, but beginning from the side and going towards the middle. Table 10-3 lists some root words that pertain to directional terms.

Table 10-3	Directional Roots
Root Word	*What It Means*
Anter/o	Front
Caud/o	Tail or downward
Cephal/o	Head or upward
Dist/o	Away from (distant) the point of origin
Dors/o	Back
Infer/o	Below
Later/o	Side
Medi/o	Middle
Poster/o	Back or behind
Proxim/o	Near to (proximity) the point of origin
Super/o	Above
Ventr/o	Front or belly

Get in position

Some frequently used anatomic positions describing body positions are

✔ **Anatomical position** is when the body is standing, arms at each side, with palms facing forward and the feet side by side. (Whether a patient is standing, or lying face up, the directional terms are always applied in the same manner.)

✔ **Erect** is standing position.

✔ **Genupectoral** is kneeling with chest resting on examining table.

✔ **Lateral recumbent** means lying on left side with right thigh and knee drawn up to chest.

✔ **Prone** means lying face down.

✔ **Supine (dorsal)** is lying flat on your back.

Regions of the Body

All of these body parts don't make a whole lot of sense until you can put them in the context of their general location within the body. Your body can be defined in several different ways, from groups and regions to cavities and planes.

Body *regions*, like the directional terms and anatomical planes we cover later, are used to specifically identify a body area. To illustrate all that's involved with a body region, take a closer look at two major regions: the abdominal and spinal.

The *abdominal area* is divided further into anatomic regions to diagnose abdominal problems with greater accuracy.

Starting with the diaphragm, which is the muscle separating the thoracic cavity from the abdominal cavity, down to the level of the pelvis or groin, the abdominal area is divided into nine equal regions.

Visualize the abdomen divided into nine squares: three across the top, three across the middle, and three across the bottom, like a tic-tac-toe board. The center portion is the *umbilical* region, the region of the navel or the umbilicus. Directly above this is the *epigastric* region, or the region of the stomach. Directly below the umbilical region is the *hypogastric* region.

On either side of the epigastric region are the *right and left hypochondriac* regions. To the right and left of the umbilical region are the *right and left lumbar regions*. To the right and left of the hypogastric region are the *right and left iliac regions*.

The anatomical divisions of the abdomen are referenced in anatomy textbooks to specify where certain organs are found.

The clinical regions of the abdomen are used to describe the abdomen when a patient is being examined. The clinical regions of the abdomen divide the abdominal area, as above, into four equal quadrants:

- ✔ **The right upper quadrant (RUQ)** contains the right lobe of the liver, gallbladder, and parts of the small and large intestines.

- ✔ **The left upper quadrant (LUQ)** contains the left lobe of the liver, stomach, pancreas, spleen, and parts of the small and large intestines.

- ✔ **The right lower quadrant (RLQ)** contains parts of the small and large intestines, appendix, right ureter, right ovary, and fallopian tube.

- ✔ **The left lower quadrant (LLQ)** contains parts of the small and large intestines, left ureter, left ovary, and fallopian tube.

Table 10-4 provides a quick look at some of the smaller body regions, beginning at the head and moving downward.

Table 10-4	Small But Mighty Body Regions
Region	*Where It Is*
Auricular region	Around the ears
Axillary	Axillae (armpits)
Buccal	Cheeks of the face
Clavicular	On each side of the sternum (breastbone)
Infraorbital	Below the eyes
Infrascapular	On each side of the chest, down to the last rib
Interscapular	On the back, between *scapulae* (shoulder blades)
Lumbar	Below the infrascapular area
Mammary	Breast area
Mental	Region of the chin
Orbital	Around the eyes
Pubic	Above the *hypogastric region* (above the pubis)
Sacral	Area over the sacrum
Sternal	Over the sternum
Submental	Below the chin
Supraclavicular	Above the clavicles

More body divisions are the regions of the spinal column, also known as the back. Note the difference between the spinal column (the *vertebrae*) and the spinal cord (the nerves running through the column). The *spinal column* is made of bone tissue, and the *spinal cord* is composed of nerve tissue.

The spinal column is divided into five regions. Begin at the top and work downward:

- ✔ **The cervical region (abbreviation C)** is located in the neck region. There are seven cervical vertebrae, C1 to C7.

- ✔ **The thoracic or dorsal region (abbreviation T or D)** is located in the chest region. There are 12 thoracic or dorsal vertebrae, T1 to T12, or D1 to D12. Each bone in this segment is joined to a rib.

- ✔ **The lumbar region (abbreviation L)** is located at the loin or the flank area between the ribs and the hip bone. There are five lumbar vertebrae, L1 to L5.

- ✔ **The sacral region (abbreviation S)** has five bones, S1 to S5, that are fused to form one bone, the *sacrum*.

- ✔ **The coccygeal region** includes the coccyx, or tailbone, a small bone composed of four fused pieces.

It is important to remember that all these terms are for directional purposes only. They provide a road map to the body. In a medical examination, directional planes, regions of the abdomen, and divisions of the spinal column are used often by the physician.

Chapter 11

All Systems Go: When Systems Combine

*T*eamwork is the key for your body systems. When they all do their own individual jobs, they have a better chance of working together in harmony. Not every single system works with every other system, but many do work together to keep you running at your top performance.

Anatomical Systems Working Together

Start with anatomy. *Anatomy* is the study of the parts of the body, from what you can see on the outside, like the skin covering muscles and bones, to the brain in the skull, or the variety of organs neatly arranged inside the trunk or torso of the body like a well-packed suitcase. Coupled with physiology (which we cover later), a bit of studying your basic building blocks will help you identify and create tons of medical terms.

A good start to learning about anatomy and physiology is to observe the body as a whole. Parts III and IV of this book cover these systems in detail, but to whet your appetite let's do a quick preview of the systems of the body.

The musculoskeletal system

The *musculoskeletal system* is made up of 206 bones and more than 600 muscles. The bones of the skeleton have tons of jobs. They provide support for the body's framework and protect vital internal organs, brain, and spinal column. Bones store minerals necessary for growth, and red bone marrow makes blood cells. Most importantly, bones make movement possible, providing attachments for muscles.

Bones are attached to other bones by *ligaments*, whereas *tendons* connect bones to muscles. A *joint* is where two bones meet.

Muscles attach to bone, not only making movement possible but holding the bones of the skeleton together. Muscles allow flexibility of the body and help maintain body temperature. But think about some other functions of muscles. There are all kinds of muscles you probably don't think too much about. Cardiac muscle keeps your heart beating, but the cardiac muscle is *involuntary*. That means you don't have to think about keeping your heart beating. Muscle contraction throughout the body keeps the blood flow moving. The digestive system is lined by smooth muscle that keeps the food moving. And don't forget the muscles that keep the bladder and colon closed up — until you voluntarily relax these muscles when you want.

The integumentary system

The *integumentary* system is a really fancy way of referring to the skin, hair, nails, and glands. The skin is actually the body's largest organ (yes, it is an organ!). It covers about 20 square feet and accounts for nearly 15 percent of your body weight. Skin (obviously) provides an external covering for the body. As a protective membrane, it prevents loss of water, salt, and heat.

The skin provides a protective barrier against bacteria, pathogens, and toxins that want to invade your body. Plus, it's full of glands that do many smaller, but equally important jobs. *Sebaceous* glands secrete oil to lubricate, whereas *sudoriferous* glands secrete sweat, acting as a cooling system. Nerves are involved as well and carry impulses that act as receptors for pain, temperature, and touch. The blood vessels in the skin aid in regulating body temperature.

The sensory system

The eyes and the ears, like the skin, are sense organs. They act as the body's external perception/alarm system by letting in light and sound. Impulses from the eyes are sent to the *occipital lobe* in the brain for processing, and impulses from the ears go to the brain's *temporal lobe*. In these lobes of the brain, nerve impulses are translated into sound sensations and visual images that we experience as vision and hearing.

Age sure takes its toll on the eyes and ears. *Presbyopia* is impaired vision due to aging. *Presbycusis* is hearing loss occurring in old age.

Physiology Systems Working Together

Physiology is the study of the function or day-to-day operation of the parts of the body. This includes the functions of everything from the smallest cell, seen only under a microscope, to a large organ like the heart. You might think that each body part has one function to carry out and works independently on its own to accomplish this function, but in fact, most body parts are team players that work together to accomplish a task. Brisk walking, for example, not only requires the use of leg muscles, but also good lung capacity to keep up the pace. You know that the heart pumps blood through the body via arteries and veins, which are part of the cardiovascular system. Without the lungs performing their function to re-oxygenate the blood as it passes through the lungs, the exchange of gases (the function of the respiratory system) would not happen, and body cells and organs would die.

Pathology (sometimes *pathophysiology*) is the study of the effects of disease on body parts and the ways disease can interfere with an organ or system's functioning ability.

The cardiovascular and lymphatic systems

The *cardiovascular system* (sometimes called the *circulatory system*) has many functions. Blood carries oxygen, nutrients, hormones, and lymph fluid to cells and transports waste products, carbon dioxide, and urea away to be excreted. The heart is the body's pumping station that pumps out freshly oxygenated blood through a vast network of vessels. The heart is divided into four chambers: two upper chambers (the *right atrium* and *left atrium* (plural: *atria*) and two lower chambers, the *right and left ventricles*.

The cardiovascular system could not survive without the assistance of the muscular system — the *myocardium* is the heart muscle — which in turn is kept functional by the *autonomic* section of the nervous system.

Not to be forgotten as a team player with the cardiovascular system is the *lymphatic system*. This system works together with the blood to fight disease. It looks after the body's immune system. This system produces *lymph*, a fluid released into the body through lymphatic vessels, which are linked up with blood vessels to carry lymph throughout the body. This system produces *lymphocytes*, the disease-fighting cells that circulate the body through blood. *Lymph nodes* located throughout the body act as the filtrating centers. Lymph nodes can trap and filter toxic and malignant substances. Special cells can digest foreign substances as well as manufacture antibodies to fight off infection.

The spleen, tonsils, and thymus are accessory organs of this system, all playing special roles. The *spleen* stores red blood cells, which can be released into the body as needed. The *thymus* gland produces lymphoctes, the disease fighters. The *tonsils* are also made up of lymphatic tissue and act as a filter system for bacteria.

The respiratory system

The *respiratory system* provides the mechanisms that allow you to breathe. You can't live without it, and, as with the other systems, improper functioning would render you dead! Now that would really ruin your day.

A fantastic voyage

Freshly oxygenated blood is pumped from the left ventricle through the *aorta* (the largest artery) into arteries that decrease in size to *arterioles* and to *capillaries*, the smallest branches of the venous system, where the exchange of gases takes place. Oxygen is absorbed into tissue cells, while carbon dioxide is expelled by the cells. The oxygen-depleted blood is carried via *venules* (small veins) through *veins*, to the *superior and inferior venae cavae*, the body's largest veins, back to the heart, where it is received in the right atrium.

But this blood has to be oxygenated before it begins the trip again, so the right atrium sends the stale blood to the right ventricle, where it then gets side-tracked to the lungs to be topped up with oxygen. The blood travels through a vast network of vessels once again, this time through *alveoli* (the air sacs of the lung), where the lungs perform the function of re-oxygenating the blood, getting it ready for its next trip around the body. Through the processes of *inspiration* and *expiration* in the lungs, fresh oxygen enters the bloodstream, and the not-needed carbon dioxide is eliminated by the lungs. This freshly oxygenated blood then comes back to the heart and is received in the left atrium, then on to the left ventricle, where it is pumped through the aorta to begin the trip all over again. Imagine this happening with every heart beat 100,000 times a day, resulting in 1,800 gallons of blood being circulated on a daily basis!

The respiratory system works in conjunction with the cardiovascular system to provide the exchange of oxygen and carbon dioxide between the air in the lungs and the blood. Inhaling and exhaling, the movement of air in and out of the lungs (*ventilation*) allows the body to maintain its oxygen requirements for body cells and tissue to survive. The lungs facilitate the exchange of oxygen and carbon dioxide between the blood and the body cells. This system also metabolizes oxygen, resulting in carbon dioxide production in body cells. Air, which is about 15 percent oxygen, enters the nose (sometimes the mouth, as in chronic mouth breathers when sleeping) — where it is moistened and warmed — through to the *pharynx* (throat), consisting of the *nasopharynx*, *oropharynx*, and *hypopharynx*.

Ventilation (breathing) is a process that again is looked after automatically by the nervous system. You don't have to consciously think about breathing. When you breathe in (*inspiration*), all passageways are opened to allow the air entry. The *diaphragm*, a large muscle separating the chest cavity from the abdominal cavity, pushes down and the ribs move up to give the lungs lots of room to expand. Air pressure within the lungs decreases and air comes in. When you breathe out (*expiration*) the diaphragm moves up, the rib cage comes down, lung pressure increases, and air is pushed out.

The lungs are contained in the *thoracic cavity* that divides into the pleural and mediastinum cavities. The *pleural cavity* surrounds the lungs, and the *mediastinal cavity* between the lungs holds the heart, trachea, and esophagus. The right lung consists of three *lobes*, and the left lung two lobes. The cavities are the *pleural* and *mediastinum*, but when referring to the area in general you should say *mediastinal cavity*, even though the area is referred to as the mediastinum.

The gastrointestinal system

The *gastrointestinal system* (also called the *digestive system* or *alimentary tract*) has three functions: to digest food, absorb nutrients, and carry waste materials to be eliminated. Except for the processes of swallowing food and having a bowel movement, what happens in between pretty much looks after itself.

We chew food, which we swallow, that goes into the esophagus and then into the stomach. The stomach partially digests the food before it moves on to the *small intestine* (also called small bowel) for further digestion and absorption. The residual food moves into the *large intestine* (large bowel) where it is doomed to be eliminated as solid waste. Except for the pharynx (throat) and esophagus, all gastrointestinal organs are in the abdominal cavity, often referred to as the *gut* or *belly*.

You've got connections

The *hypopharynx* is a common passageway for both food and air to travel to their final destinations. Air taken through the nose to the larynx produces the voice. The *trachea* (windpipe) connects the larynx to a right and left *bronchus*, just above the lungs. The bronchi break down into smaller branches called *bronchioles* that lead into small clusters resembling grapes.

These grape-like sacs are called *alveoli*, of which there are approximately 300 million in healthy lungs, surrounded in *capillaries*. Oxygen moves from alveoli into the lung capillaries surrounding them to be exchanged via the bloodstream throughout the body. Carbon dioxide moves from the capillaries into the alveoli to be expelled by the lungs.

The accessory organs of this system — teeth, salivary glands, liver, gallbladder, and pancreas — all do their special part to add in the process of digestion, absorption, and elimination. The pancreas (also part of the endocrine system) secretes *enzymes* necessary for digestion. The liver (the body's largest gland) secretes *bile* needed for digestion. It metabolizes proteins, fats, and carbohydrates. The liver also acts as a filter system that neutralizes toxins. The gallbladder stores bile that also aids the digestive process.

The liver joins a group of mixed-function organs (working as both organ and gland) that includes the stomach, intestines, kidney, ovaries, and testes. In addition to their regular system functions, they also produce hormones.

Digested food and nutrients are absorbed into the bloodstream through the walls of the small intestine, so blood and the cardiovascular systems again assist another system. All the while, the muscular system provides the *peristalsis*, a wave-like contractions of muscle throughout this long tract of passageways, that propels the food onward and outward.

This system is very prone to inflammation because of the invasion of foreign material (food). Food poisoning is a perfect example, but let's not forget *gastroenteritis* (inflammation of stomach and intestines), vomiting, and everyone's favorite, *diarrhea*.

The endocrine system

The *endocrine system* maintains the chemical balance in the body. It works in conjunction with the nervous system to regulate body systems. This is accomplished by sending messengers called *hormones* through the body via the bloodstream. The nervous system controls the endocrine system's release of hormones, and hormones control the *metabolic* function in the body. The *pituitary gland*, known as the "master gland," is located in the brain. It works together with the *hypothalamus gland* to aid homeostasis and body functions such as growth, salt and water balance, reproduction, and metabolism.

Homeostasis is an automatic process that maintains stability and balance of the body's internal environment in order to stay healthy.

Glands that make up this system include the thyroid, parathyroids, adrenals, and pineal. All these glands produce hormones. The *pancreas* (also a part of the digestive system) also produces hormones. The pancreas joins a group of mixed-function organs including the stomach, intestines, kidney, ovaries, and testes. In addition to their regular system functions, they also produce hormones.

The *thyroid gland* secretes two hormones that are necessary for the body to maintain a normal rate of metabolism. The *parathyroid glands* secrete a hormone that moves the storage of calcium from bone into the blood (to maintain adequate levels of calcium in the bloodstream).

The *adrenal glands* are made up of the cortex and medulla. The *cortex* secretes *steroids* and mineral *corticoids.* which are essential to life because they regulate the levels of mineral salts, or *electrolytes*. In fact, all adrenal hormones secreted by the cortex are steroids. These include mineralocorticoids, which regulate potassium, sodium and chloride (electrolytes) and glucocorticoids (which includes cortisol) that aids in metabolism of carbohydrates, fat and proteins (tissues release glucose to raise blood sugar levels when needed).

The *adrenal medulla* secretes catecholamines only, such as epinephrine (adrenaline) and norepinephrine (noradrenaline), which aid the body in stressful situations.

The pancreas has specialized cells called the *islets of Langerhans*. They produce insulin and *glucagon,* which stimulates *gluconeogenesis*, or sugar production, in the liver. *Insulin* is necessary in the blood so sugar can pass from the blood into cells. The *pineal gland* secretes melatonin, thought to affect the brain, help regulate sleep patterns, and influence the rate of gonad maturation.

The endocrine glands all play a part in this large orchestra to maintain the harmonious music of the body. The hypothalamus and pituitary are the orchestra leaders of this complex system, which needs to function properly to maintain good health.

The three little systems

The *central nervous system* includes the brain and spinal cord. The *peripheral nervous system* consists of *cranial* and *spinal nerves*, or all the nerves that branch out from the brain and spinal cord. Impulses are sent to and from the brain via a vast network of nerves. The peripheral system consists of nerves that operate automatically, sending impulses from the central nervous system to glands, the heart, and blood vessels as well as the involuntary muscles in the digestive and urinary systems. This autonomic system also contains sympathetic nerves that stimulate the body when under stress or in a crisis, to increase blood pressure and heart rate.

The nervous system

The *nervous system* is one of the most complicated systems in the body. More than 10 *billion* nerve cells function constantly to organize and coordinate the activities of the body. This system controls voluntary as well as involuntary functions. We speak, move muscles, hear, taste, see, and think. We have memory, a word bank, association, and discrimination. These enormous tasks represent just a small number of functions controlled by the nervous system.

The brain controls *homeostasis*, an automatic checklist your body goes through, to keep all systems running normally. When the body is stressed due to infection, pain, or not enough oxygen, body cells are not at their best and don't function as well as they should. So the brain monitors blood pressure, body temperature, and sugar in the blood. The *hypothalamus*, located in the brain, maintains homeostasis by initiating the release of hormones when needed.

Most major regions of your body host some sort of nervous system worker bee, from your head to your toes.

- The brain's largest part is the *cerebrum*. The lobes of the cerebrum control functions such as speech, recognizing objects, concentration, vision, problem solving, hearing, learning, and almost all functions of consciousness,

- The *cerebellum*, or "hind brain," assists in coordinating voluntary body movement and helps maintain body balance. The hypothalamus controls body temperature, sleep, and appetite.

- The *medulla oblongata* regulates the centers that control respiration, heart rate, and the respiratory system.

- The *spinal cord* passes through the *vertebral canal* from the *medulla* down to the *lumbar vertebrae*. The cord conducts nerve impulses to and from the brain.

You can see why the nervous system is so complex. It is the body's control center, and the spinal cord with its nerve network is the body's communication system.

The urinary and reproductive systems

Think you're running out of systems? Not a chance! Next, consider your urinary system, whose responsibility it is to remove the liquid waste from the body. *Urine* is liquid waste filtered from the blood, collected in the *tubules* of the kidneys, and passed along to the *renal pelvis*, the central collecting portion of each of two kidneys, down each *ureter* (we each have two) to the *urinary bladder*, which is, of course, the holding tank. When urination occurs, urine is released from the bladder, travels down the urethra, and exits the body.

Much of this system also looks after itself automatically. It works in conjunction with the bloodstream to begin the filtration process with the autonomic nervous system, so we don't have to *think* about producing urine, we only have to release it when the bladder is full. The muscular system involves the *sphincter* that we control to open to release urine from the body.

The kidneys play an important role in the process of homeostasis — to keep everything in sync and in order. Kidneys help maintain the proper balance of salt and water content in the blood as well as maintain the proper acid-base balance in the blood. The kidneys work together with the liver and adrenal glands to maintain balance of sodium and potassium in the blood, which affects blood volume and, in turn, affects blood pressure. Once again, this is an example of multiple systems working together to accomplish an important task.

In the male, the *prostate* surrounds the urethra. The urethra passes through the prostate as its connection to the male reproductive system. During urination, urine passes through the male urethra.

During ejaculation, *seminal fluid* passes through the urethra, so the urethra serves two purposes in the male. The *prostate gland* secretes juices that help make up the seminal fluid.

The reproductive systems have one purpose: to secrete hormones (accomplished through the endocrine system) in order to have the ability to reproduce. To accomplish this, a male must fertilize a female, either in person or via one of the many modern fertility clinical procedures.

The female system consists of the *ovaries* (the *gonads*) that produce the hormones *estrogen* and *progesterone*. The *fallopian tube* is the passageway that a mature *ovum* (egg) takes from the ovary to the uterus. The *uterus* is a muscular, very expandable organ that provides a safe place for a pregnancy to grow to maturity (40 weeks). The *vagina* is the birth canal, the route taken by the infant at delivery and also the route taken by the sperm to achieve the pregnancy. Actually, fertilization of a sperm and an ovum takes place in the fallopian tube and then travels to the uterus to grow. Each month the uterus prepares for a possible pregnancy. When conception does not occur, the lining of the uterus is expelled as a *menstrual period*. Then the whole monthly process begins all over again.

The breasts are considered part of the reproductive system as they are the glands that begin producing milk following delivery.

In the male, the *testes* are the gonads. It is in the testes or *testicles*, which are held in the *scrotum*, that the hormone *testosterone* is produced, as well as *spermatozoa*, which are stored in the *epididymis*. At the time of ejaculation, the spermatozoa together with seminal fluid gathered along the route, travels through a duct system that includes the *vas deferens, seminal vesicles,* prostate, and urethra, via the penis, to exit the body. During intercourse, it is all deposited into the vagina.

We're sure you'll agree that, when all is said and done, the human body is a pretty amazing machine!

Part III
In Terms of Anatomy

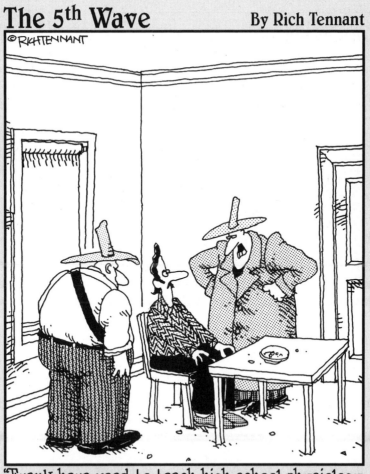

The 5th Wave   By Rich Tennant

"Frank here used to teach high school physiology,
so if you value your Zygomatic arch or your
Alveolar margins, you'll start talking."

In this part . . .

*I*n this part, you get down and dirty with your anatomy and learn more terms than you thought possible. Chapter 12 familiarizes you with the skeletal system, while Chapter 13 pumps you up with information about the muscular system. Chapter 14 delves into all of your extras like hair, skin, and nails. And Chapter 15 takes you on a journey of the senses and their appropriate terms.

Chapter 12

Boning Up on the Skeletal System

Consider the skeletal system to be your body's infrastructure. This system, along with its joints, works together with the muscles to give your body the support it needs to function. The bony skeleton, composed of 206 bones, provides the jointed framework for the body, giving it shape. This framework protects vital organs from external injury and provides attachment points for muscles, ligaments, and tendons to make body movement possible.

Bones are connected to other bones by ligaments. Muscles are connected to bones by tendons, which are located at each end of a muscle because a muscle needs to be attached to two bones to make movement possible. A joint, then, is any place in the body where two or more bones meet.

How the Skeletal System Works

Although bones, muscles, joints, ligaments, and tendons all work together, they each have a special job. Bones provide framework but ligaments and tendons provide the attachments for muscles to contract and relax.

Bones store mineral salts, and the inner core of a bone is composed of *hematopoietic* (blood cell forming) red bone marrow. Other areas of the bone are used as storage areas for minerals necessary for growth, such as calcium and phosphorus.

Red bone marrow is red because red blood cells form in it. In adults red marrow is eventually replaced by yellow marrow, which stores fat. Bones are complete organs, chiefly made up of connective tissue called *osseous* or *bony* tissue plus a rich supply of blood vessels and nerves.

Colles' fracture was first described by Dr. Andrew Colles, an Irish surgeon in 1814. It is a fracture of the distal end of the radius (*distal* meaning the portion of a body part farthest from the point of origin). But you don't have to be Irish to sustain one. In this case the point of origin is the shoulder, looking at the limb separately, and not the body as a whole.

Bones and osteology

Now it's time to get down with osteology. No, it's not a slick new dance move. *Osteology* is the study of bones. Notice the root word *osteo*? You might know it as part of the word *osteoporosis* — a common condition typical in women involving the loss of bone density. So, *osteo* is the focus in this chapter. The first step into the world of osteology is looking at the actual makeup of our bones.

Bones are classified by their shape — long, short, flat, irregular, and sesamoid.

- ✔ **Long bones,** found in arms (the *humerus* is the upper arm) and legs (the *femur* is your thigh) are strong, broad at the ends where they join with other bones, and have large surface areas for muscle attachment.
- ✔ **Short bones** are found in the wrists and ankles and have small, irregular shapes.
- ✔ **Flat bones** are found covering soft body parts. The shoulder blades, ribs, and pelvic bones are examples of flat bones.
- ✔ Vertebrae are examples of **irregular bones.**
- ✔ **Sesamoid bones** are small, rounded bones found near joints. The kneecap is an example of a sesamoid bone.

There's more to bones than the hard, white substance you think of when you envision one. For starters, the shaft or middle region of a long bone is called the *diaphysis*. Each end of a long bone is called the *epiphysis*. Both are joined by the *physis*, also called the *growth plate*. The *periosteum* of the bone is a strong, fibrous membrane that covers the surface, except at the ends. Bones other than long bones are completely covered by the periosteum.

Fractures are often classified by a system called the *Salter-Harris system*, which identifies whether a fracture involves the epiphysis, physis, diaphysis, or some combination of all three.

Beneath the periosteum is a level of *osteoblasts*, which deposit calcium and phosphorus compounds in the bony tissue. *Articular cartilage* covers the ends of long bones. This cartilage layer cushions the bones where they meet with other bones, or at the joints. The *compact bone* is made of dense tissue lying under the periosteum in all bones. Within the compact bone is a system of small channels containing blood vessels that bring oxygen and nutrients to the bone and remove waste products such as carbon dioxide.

Cancellous bone, sometimes called *spongy bone*, is more porous and less dense than compact bone. Spaces in cancellous bone contain red bone marrow, which is richly supplied with blood and consists of immature and mature blood cells in various stages of development. The ribs, the pelvic bones, the sternum or breastbone and vertebrae, as well as the epiphyses of long bones, contain red bone marrow within cancellous tissue. Figure 12-1 illustrates the skeleton.

Axial skeleton

Think of the word *axis* when you think about the axial skeleton. The bones that make up this particular part of the skeleton tend to encircle important organs or rotate in an axial motion. The axial skeleton includes the heavy hitters in this section.

Cranium

The bones of the cranium (skull) protect the brain. The bones of the skull include the *frontal bone*, which forms the forehead and bony sockets that contain the eyes. The *parietal bone* forms the roof and upper sides of the skull. Two *temporal* bones form the lower sides and base. The *mastoid process* is a small round part of the temporal bone behind the ear.

The *occipital bone* forms the back and base of the skull and joins the parietal and temporal bones, forming a *suture* (a joining line) of cranial bones. The occipital bone has an opening called the *foramen magnum* through which the spinal cord passes. The *sphenoid bone* extends behind the eyes and forms part of the base of the skull. It joins the frontal, occipital, and ethmoid bones and serves as an anchor to hold these bones together. The *ethmoid bone* is a thin delicate bone, supporting the nasal cavity and forms part of the orbits of the eyes.

Be careful when working with a newborn cranium, as the cranial bones of a newborn are not completely joined. There are gaps of *unossified* tissue (tissue that is still in the fibrous membrane stage) in the skull, called the soft spot or *fontanelle*. The lines where the bones of the skull join are called *cranial sutures*. The pulse of blood vessels can be felt under the skin in these areas.

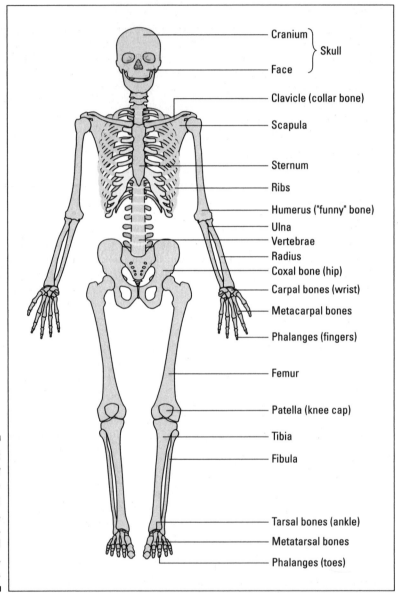

Figure 12-1:
Front view
of the skele-
ton showing
rib cage,
clavicles,
upper and
lower limbs,
and pelvis.

From LifeARTS®, Super Anatomy 1, ©2002, Lippincott Williams & Wilkins

Facial bones

All the facial bones except one are joined together. Only the *mandible*, or lower jaw bone, is capable of moving, which is necessary for chewing and speaking. Other facial bones include the *nasal* bones, and the *maxillary* bones. Two large bones compose the upper jaw. Both the mandible and maxilla contain sockets called *alveoli*, in which the teeth are embedded. The mandible joins the skull at the temporal bone, forming the lengthily named *temporomandibular joint*. The *zygoma* or *zygomatic bones* form the cheek.

Vertebral column

The *vertebral column*, or spinal column, is composed of 26 bone segments called *vertebrae* (singular *vertebra*), which are arranged in five *divisions:* cervical, thoracic, lumbar, sacrum, and coccyx (tailbone).

The first seven vertebrae are called the *cervical vertebrae* (C1-C7). These vertebrae do not join with the ribs. The first cervical vertebra, C1 (also known as the *atlas*), articulates with the occipital bone of the skull at the back of neck. It supports the head and allows it to move forward and back. The second cervical vertebra, C2 (the *axis*), acts as a pivot, about which the atlas rotates, allowing head to turn from side to side, extend, and flex.

The second division consists of 12 *thoracic vertebrae* (T1-T12). These vertebrae join with the 12 pairs of ribs. The third division consists of five *lumbar vertebrae* (L1-L5). They are the strongest and largest of the back bones. The *sacrum* is a slightly curved triangular bone, composed of five separate segments, or sacral bones, that gradually become fused. The *coccyx* is the tailbone. It is also a fused bone, formed from four small *coccygeal bones*.

The Greek *diskos* means "flat plate." An example is the lumbar disk. And coccyx comes from the Greek word for cuckoo; it resembles a cuckoo's beak.

A vertebra is composed of a disk-shaped portion called the *vertebral body*, which is the solid anterior portion (closest to body front, farthest from the body back). A *lamina* is a part of the posterior (back) portion of a vertebra. *Spinous processes*, *thoracic processes*, and *transverse processes* are little winglike projections that project or extend from each vertebra. The *foramen* is the opening in the middle of each vertebra that the spinal cord passes through.

Between the body of one vertebra and the bodies of vertebrae lying beneath, are *vertebral disks* which help to provide flexibility and cushion shock to the vertebral column.

Thorax

The thorax (not to be confused with something invented by Dr. Seuss) starts with the *clavicle,* or the collarbone, connecting the sternum (breastbone) to each shoulder. The *scapula* is the shoulder blade, consisting of two flat triangular bones, one on each back side of the thorax. The scapulae extend to join with the clavicle at the *acromion*.

The *sternum* is the breastbone, the flat bone extending down the midline of the chest. The uppermost part of the sternum joins to the sides of the clavicle and ribs, whereas the other, narrowed portion is attached to the diaphragm. The lower portion of the sternum is the *xiphoid process*, the small, mobile bone tag on the very end of the sternum. This is the thing you would feel for when placing your hands on a chest to perform CPR. The 12 pairs of ribs are close neighbors with the sternum. The first seven pair join the sternum anteriorly (at the chest) by attachments of *costal cartilage*. Ribs 1–7 are called true ribs. Ribs 8–12 are called false ribs. The false ribs join with the vertebral column in the back, but join the 7th rib anteriorly and do not attach to the sternum. Ribs 11 and 12 are called floating ribs because they are completely free at their anterior end.

Pelvis

The *pelvic girdle* or hip bone is a large bone that supports the trunk of the body and joins with the femur (thigh bone) and *sacrum*. The adult pelvic bone is composed of three pairs of fused bone: the *ilium*, the *ischium,* and the *pubis*.

The ilium is the uppermost and largest portion. The connection between the iliac bones and the sacrum is so firm that they are often referred to as one bone, the *sacroiliac*. The *iliac crests* are found on both the anterior and posterior portions of the pelvis. They are filled with red bone marrow and serve as an attachment for abdominal wall muscles.

The ischium is the posterior portion of the pelvis. The ischium and the muscles attached to it are what we sit on.

The pubis is the anterior portion containing two parts that are joined by way of a disk. This area of fusion is called the *pubic symphysis*. The region within the bone formed by the pelvic girdle is called the *pelvic cavity*. The rectum, sigmoid colon, bladder and female reproductive organs are contained in this cavity.

Appendicular skeleton

Think of the word *appendage* when your thoughts turn to the appendicular skeleton. Your reachers, grabbers, and hoofers are all covered in this section. Appendages fall into two major categories of bones.

Upper extremeties

Arms and hands are part of this category. The bones of the arm and hand include the *humerus*, the upper arm bone. The large head of the humerus is round and joins the scapula and clavicle. The *ulna* and *radius* are the bones of the lower arm or forearm. The bony prominence of the ulna at the elbow is called the *olecranon*. *Carpals* are wrist bones. Finally, there are two rows of four bones. The *metacarpals* are five bones radiating to the fingers. *Phalanges* (the singular is *phalanx*) are the finger bones.

Each finger has three phalanges: the proximal, middle, and distal. The *proximal* is the phalange closest to the point of origin, whereas the *distal* is farthest from the point of origin. So, the proximal would be the first after the knuckle, the middle would be in the middle, and the distal at the fingertip. The thumb has only two phalanges: medial and distal at tip of the thumb.

Diaphysis comes from Greek *diaphusis*, meaning "state of growing between." Diaphysis is the shaft of long bones that grows as children grow.

Leg and foot

The *femur* is the thigh bone. At the top end of it, a rounded head fits into a socket in the hip bone called the *acetabulum*. The *patella*, or kneecap, is a small flat bone that lies in front of the joint between the femur and one of the lower leg bones called the *tibia*. The tibia is the largest of the two lower bones of the leg, often referred to as the shin bone. The *fibula* is the smaller of the two bones.

The *tarsals*, or ankle bones, are short bones that are much like the carpal bones of the wrist, but larger. The *calcaneus,* the largest of these bones, is also called the heel bone. *Metatarsals* compose the forefoot or bones leading to the phalanges in the toes. There are two phalanges in the big or great toe and three in each of the other four toes. Just like the fingers, all the bones in the toes are phalanges, from proximal to distal. In the big or great toe they are called the proximal and distal, differing slightly from the thumb.

The femur is the longest bone in the body.

Joints

Now think about the "glue" that holds all these bones together. Okay, joints aren't really made of glue, but they sure do a good job of keeping everything connected. Let us articulate that concept a bit better: Joints, also called *articulations*, are the coming together of two or more bones. Some are not movable, such as the *suture joints* between the cranial bones. Some joints only partially move, such as joints between the vertebrae.

Most joints do allow movement. These freely movable joints are called *synovial joints*. An example is the ball and socket type — the hip joint, for example, in which the head of the femur fits into the acetabulum. Another synovial joint is the hinged type as seen at the elbow, knee, or ankle joints.

The bones of a synovial joint are separated by a *capsule*, composed of fibrous cartilage. Ligaments of connective tissue hold the bones together around the capsule to strengthen it. The bone surfaces at a joint are covered with a smooth surface called the *articular cartilage*. The *synovial membrane* is the inner layer of the capsule, the layer beneath the capsular surface.

The *synovial cavity* is filled with a lubricating fluid produced by synovial membranes. This fluid contains water and nutrients that help to lubricate the joints so that friction on the articular cartilage is minimal.

Bursae (singular *bursa*) are closed sacs of synovial fluid lined with synovial membrane. They lie in the spaces between tendons, ligaments, and bones and lubricate areas where friction would normally develop close to the joint capsule. The *olecranon bursa* at the elbow joint and the *patellar bursa* at the knee are examples of bursae.

Skeletal Root Words

Now that you've gotten to know the specific parts of the skeletal system a bit better, it's time to put your expertise into practice by breaking down the root words into meanings and useful applications. The roots, as always, are essential medical terminology knowledge because once you master these roots (those good ol' Greek and Latin ones, that is), you can break down any skeletal-related word and discover its meaning.

Table 12-1 lists important skeletal system root words and combining forms.

Table 12-1	Digging Up Your Skeletal Roots
Root Word	**What It Means**
Kyph/o	Humpback (posterior curvature of thoracic spine)
Lamin/o	Lamina (part of the vertebral arch)
Lord/o	Curve or swayback (*lordosis*: anterior curvature in lumbar spine)
Lumb/o	Lower back, lumbar region
Myel/o	Bone marrow
Oste/o	Bone
Orth/o	Straight
Scoli/o	Crooked, bent (scoliosis: lateral curvature of spine)
Spondyl/o	Vertebra (referring to conditions of the structure)
Vertebr/o	Vertebra (referring to describing the structure)

Table 12-2 lists the combining forms used with bones.

Table 12-2	Bone-related Combining Forms	
Combining Form	**Example**	**What It Means**
Acetabul/o	Acetabulum	Hip joint
Calcane/o	Cancaneus	Heel
Carp/o	Carpals	Wrist bones
Clavic/o, clavicul/o	Clavicle	Collar bone
Cost/o	Costal	Ribs
Crani/o	Cranium	Skull
Femor/o	Femur	Upper leg bone
Fibul/o	Fibula	Lower leg bone
Humer/o	Humerus	Upper arm bone
Ili/o	Ilium	Pelvic bone
Ischi/o	Ischium	Pelvic bone
Lumb/o	Spine	Lumbar region
Malleol/o	Malleolus	Ankle
Mandibul/o	Mandible	Lower jaw
Maxill/o	Maxilla	Upper jaw

(continued)

Table 12-2 (continued)

Combining Form	Example	What It Means
Metacarp/o	Metacarpals	Bones of hand
Metatars/o	Metatarsals	Bones of foot
Olecran/o	Olecranon	Elbow
Patell/o	Patella	Knee cap
Phalang/o	Phalanges	Bones of fingers and toes
Pub/o	Pubis	Portion of pelvic bone
Radi/o	Radius	Lower arm bone
Sacr/o	Sacrum	Sacral area of spine
Scapul/o	Scapula	Shoulder blade
Stern/o	sternum	Breastbone
Tars/o	Tarsals	Ankle bones
Tibi/o	Tibia	Lower leg bone
Uln/o	Ulna	Lower arm bone

Table 12-3 lists the combining forms used with joints.

Table 12-3   Joint-related Combining Forms

Combining Form	What It Means
Arthr/o	Joint
Articul/o	Joint
Burs/o	Bursa
Chondr/o	Cartilage
Disk/o	Intervertebral disk
Fibros/o	Fibrous
Menisc/o	Meniscus
Synovi/o	Synovium
Ten/o, tend/o, tendin/o	Tendon

More Anatomical Terms

Although the makeup of the skeletal system is pretty straightforward, there are still more useful terms you need to know in order to communicate about 'dem bones. Try a few of the words in Table 12-4 on for size.

Table 12-4	More Common Skeletal Vocabulary
Word	*What It Means*
Ankylosis	Stiffness of a joint
Arthralgia	Pain in the joint
Articulation	Joint
Bradykinesia	Slow movement
Bursa	Sac of fluid at or around a joint
Calcium	One of the mineral constituents of bone
Cancellous bone	Spongy porous bone tissue
Chiropodist	Specialist in diagnosing and treating foot disorders
Chiropractics	System of therapy that consists of manipulation of the vertebral column
Chiropractor	Specialist in chiropractics
Chondromalacia	Softening of cartilage
Compact bone	Hard, dense bone tissue
Condyle	Knuckle-like process at the end of a bone – near a joint
Diaphysis	Shaft or midportion of a long bone
Dyskinesia	Difficult movement
Dystrophy	Abnormal development
Epiphysis	End of a long bone
Fissure	Narrow slit-like opening between bones
Fontanelle	Soft spot, incomplete closure of infant's skull sutures
Fossa	Depression or cavity in a bone
Hematopoiesis	Development of blood cells in bone marrow
Hyperkinesia	Excessive movement or overactivity
Intercostal	Between the ribs
Intracranial	Within the cranium
Kyphosis	Abnormal hump of thoracic spine, "hunchback"
Ligament	Connective tissue binding bones to other bones
Mastoid process	Round projection on the temporal bone behind the ear
Orthopedics	Branch of medicine dealing with the study and treatment of diseases and abnormalities of the skeletal system
Orthopedist	Physician specializing in orthopedics
Orthotics	Making and fitting of orthopedic appliances such as arch supports, used to support, align, or correct deformities

(continued)

Table 12-4 *(continued)*

Word	What It Means
Osseous tissue	Bone tissue
Ossification	Process of bone formation
Osteoblast	A bone cell that helps form bone tissue
Osteoclast	A bone cell that absorbs and removes unwanted bone tissue
Osteopath	Physician who specializes in osteopathy
Osteopathy	Branch of medicine using the usual forms of diagnosis of treatment but with emphasis on the role of the relationship between the body organs and the skeletal system, and performing manipulations in order to decrease pain and help body function
Osteosarcoma	Malignant tumor of bone
Podiatrist	Specialist in diagnosing and treating foot disorders such as corns and ingrown toenails; some also perform foot surgery
Prosthesis	Artificial substitute or replacement for a missing body part such as an artificial leg, eye, joint, or heart valve
Red bone marrow	Found in cancellous bone, the site of hematopoiesis
Scoliosis	Abnormal lateral curvature of the spine
Subcostal	Below the ribs
Tendinitis or tendonitis	Inflammation of a tendon
Tendon	Connective tissue binding muscles to bones
Tenodynia	Pain in a tendon
Tenosynovitis	Inflammation of the tendon and synovial membrane
Trabeculae	Supporting bundles of bony fibers in cancellous or sponge bone
Trochanter	Large process behind the neck of the femur
Tubercle	Small rounded process on a bone
Tuberosity	Large rounded process on a bone
Yellow bone marrow	The fatty tissue found in the diaphyses of long bones

Common Skeletal Conditions

Breaks, sprains, and bunions are no fun. Many of the most common maladies associated with the skeletal system involve the application of casts or other corrective devices. Good, old-fashioned *fractures* (a sudden break of the bone) top the list of skeletal conditions. Whether a result of an auto accident or just plain clumsiness (come on, like you didn't see that curb jump out at you!), any bone in your body is a potential break waiting to happen.

You are probably familiar with many common bone conditions because you've likely experienced one of them.

- ✔ **Bunion** is an abnormal prominence with bursal swelling at the metatarsophalangeal joint near the base of the big toe.

- ✔ **Bursitis** is an inflammation of a bursa. Tennis elbow is an example of bursitis of the olecranon bursa.

- ✔ **Dislocation** is a displacement of a bone from its joint. Dislocations may be reduced or restored to their normal condition and the joint immobilized with sling or strapping for healing of torn ligaments and tendons.

- ✔ **Sprain**, everyone's favorite, is trauma or injury to a joint with pain, swelling, and injury to ligaments.

Break it to me gently, Doc

Don't think every fracture is a run-of-the-mill break. You'd be surprised at how complicated a fracture can be. Here's a sampling from the fracture menu:

- ✔ **Closed fracture:** Bone is broken with no open wound in the skin.

- ✔ **Comminuted fracture:** Bone is splintered, crushed, or completely detached.

- ✔ **Compression fracture:** Bone is compressed; occurring in the vertebrae.

- ✔ **Greenstick fracture:** Bone is partially bent and partially broken, like when a green stick breaks. Often occurs in children.

- ✔ **Impacted fracture:** Bone is broken with one end wedged into the other.

- ✔ **Open (compound) fracture:** Broken bone with an open skin wound.

Treatment of fractures includes *reduction*, restoring the fracture to its normal position. There are two types of reduction:

- ✔ **Closed reduction** involves a manipulated reduction without an incision.

- ✔ **Open reduction** features an incision into the fracture site to restore normal position.

Once the fractured bone is set, a fiberglass or plaster of Paris cast, which is a solid mold of the body part, is applied to the injured area while healing takes place.

Possibly the most painful is the *protrusion of an intervertebral disk*, an abnormal extension of the intervertebral pad into the neural canal. This is commonly referred to as a *herniated disk* or *slipped disk*.

The bones can also experience conditions due to deformity and growths. *Talipes*, also known as clubfoot, is a congenital deformity of the bones of the foot. The bones are twisted out of shape or position. *Exostoses* are bony growths (benign tumors) on the surface of a bone.

Let's not forget our old friend, *arthritis*, the inflammation of a joint. Speaking of old, this condition is not limited to seniors. Arthritis knows no age, and it has several permutations:

- **Ankylosing spondylitis** is a chronic arthritis with stiffening of joints, particularly the spine. This condition responds to corticosteroids and anti-inflammatory therapy.

- **Gouty arthritis (gout)** is inflammation of joints caused by excessive uric acid in the body. An inherited defect in metabolism causes excessive uric acid to accumulate in the blood, joints, and soft tissues near the joints. Gout commonly occurs in the big (great) toe.

- **Osteoarthritis** is chronic inflammation of bones and joints due to degenerative changes in the cartilage. This occurs mainly in the hips and legs. Drug therapy reduces the inflammation and pain, and physical therapy loosens impaired joints.

- **Rheumatoid arthritis** is a chronic disease where joints become inflamed and painful. In rheumatoid arthritis, the small joints of the hands and feet are usually affected first, and the larger joints later.

Finding the Culprit: Skeletal Diseases and Pathology

Some conditions affecting the skeletal system are more complicated and are considered *pathological* diseases, which are diseases that occur because of structural or functional changes caused by a disease. Some may sound familiar to you, including *osteoporosis*, a decrease in bone density due to loss of calcium. Osteoporosis may occur as part of the aging process or due to corticosteroid therapy.

Two other diseases with the *osteo-* root are *osteomyelitis* and *osteogenic sarcoma*. The former is an inflammation of the bone and bone marrow due to infection. Bacteria enters the body through a wound, spreads from an infection near the bone, or originates in a skin or throat infection. Infection occurs in the long bones of the arm and leg, which can lead to an abscess and, if the bone dies, a *sequestrum* (a segment of dead bone) may develop. *Osteogenic sarcoma* is a malignant tumor of bone. Similarly, *Ewing's tumor* is a highly malignant metastasizing tumor (Ewing's sarcoma) involving the entire shaft of a long bone. It occurs in children and adolescents.

Most lesions associated with osteogenic sarcoma occur just above or below the knee.

Inflammation is not just for muscles and soft tissues. Bones can become inflamed as well. *Rickets* is inflammation of the spinal column, characterized by *osteomalacia* or softening of bone. It is a disease of infancy and childhood when bones that are forming fail to receive the calcium and phosphorus they need. Bones become soft and bend easily.

Rickets and osteogenic sarcoma are most common in childhood.

Testing, Testing: Skeletal Radiology and Diagnostic Tests

X-rays of bones and joints are common procedures to identify fractures or tumors, to monitor healing of a fracture, and to identify abnormal structures. The major methods to the skeletal madness are as follows:

- ✔ **Arthrocentesis:** Surgical puncture of a joint to aspirate fluid for diagnostic purposes

- ✔ **Arthrogram:** X-ray film of a joint

- ✔ **Arthroscopy:** Visual examination of the interior of a joint using an arthroscope

- ✔ **Bone densitometry (bone density):** Determines the density of bone, performed to diagnose osteoporosis

- ✔ **Bone scan (nuclear medicine test):** Detects presence of metastatic disease of the bone and monitors degenerative bone disease

- ✔ **Computerized tomography (CT):** Gives accurate definition of bone structure and can demonstrate even slight changes

- ✔ **Fluoroscopy:** Examination using a fluoroscope, a device used to examine deep body structures by means of X-rays

- ✔ **Magnetic resonant imaging (MRI):** Evaluates all soft tissues and is especially useful for assessing the ligaments, tendons, muscles, spinal stenosis, and degenerative disk changes; great for anything that doesn't show up on an X-ray

- ✔ **Single-photon emission computerized tomography (SPECT):** A very sensitive nuclear method for detecting bone abnormalities

Paging Dr. Terminology: Skeletal Surgeries and Procedures

Both bones and joints can be repaired with surgery. Joints can be surgically fixed with *arthrodesis* or surgically repaired with *arthroplasty*. There are three types of arthroplasties:

- ✔ **Total hip replacement arthroplasty** is performed for degenerative joint disease or arthritis. The surgery involves replacement of the head of the femur of the hip joint with a prosthetic (artificial) metallic femoral head and a plastic-coated replacement *acetabulum* (a cup that the femoral head fits into).

- ✔ **Total knee joint replacement arthroplasty** is performed to replace worn surfaces of the knee joint. Various prostheses are used in this procedure.

- ✔ **Metatarsal arthroplasty** is performed to treat deformities associated with rheumatoid arthritis or *hallux valgus* (a deformity of the big toe), and to treat painful or unstable joints.

Remember the root *arthro* when discussing joints. Arthritis is the inflammation of a joint, and most of the surgical procedures for joints use the same root *arthro*.

The lone exception to the *arthro* rule is *synovectomy*, which is the excision of synovial membrane of a joint.

The head and spine have several surgical options. A *craniotomy*, an incision into the skull, allows access to the brain for surgery. A *diskectomy* is an excision of an intervertebral disk. On the other hand, a *percutaneous diskectomy* is a procedure that uses fluoroscopy to guide insertion of a Nucleotome into a spinal disk, to remove the thick, sticky nucleus of the disk. *Nucleotome* is a registered brand name for instruments and protocol used to perform an automated percutaneous lumbar diskectomy. This allows the disk to soften and contract, relieving the lower back and leg pain. The excision of a lamina relieves symptoms of a ruptured disk, and a *spondylosyndesis* is the fusing together of the vertebrae (spinal fusion). A *lamina* is a part of the posterior (back) portion of a vertebra.

Don't forget about fixing the appendicular skeleton (remember those good old appendages?). Fixing an arm or leg bone is about more than wrapping it in a cast. Consider these surgical options:

- **Meniscectomy:** Excision of a meniscus for a torn cartilage in the knee
- **Osteoclasis:** Surgical breaking of a bone to correct a deformity
- **Osteoplasty:** Surgical repair of a bone
- **Osteotomy:** Incision into a bone
- **Patellectomy:** Excision of the patella
- **Tenorrhaphy:** Suturing of a tendon
- **Tenotomy:** Incision of a tendon

Chapter 13

Getting Ripped: The Muscular System

In This Chapter

▶ Finding out how your muscular system works

▶ Determining root words, prefixes, and suffixes appropriate to this system

▶ Using terminology of the muscular system to discuss common conditions and diseases

▶ Finding the right terms to use when diagnosing problems

*T*hink about this the next time you hit the gym: Your body is the proud owner of more than 600 muscles! Luckily, you don't have to pump a different weight machine to work every single one. The beauty of the muscular system is that it is, in fact, a system in which different major muscle groups work together at the same time.

So relax and don't stress too much about that rowing machine. You're using muscles right now reading this book.

How the Muscular System Works

The *musculoskeletal* system is made up of muscles and joints. The muscles — all 600 of them and more — are responsible for movement. The skeleton provides attachment points and support for muscles, but it's the muscle tissue's ability to extend and contract that makes movement happen. So, for every climb of the elliptical machine, you can thank muscular tissue for making it possible.

Muscles make up the major part of fleshy portions of the body and account for one half of body weight. Muscles vary in proportion to body size, and the shape of the body is determined by muscles covering bones.

Tendons: The ultimate wingmen

You've gotta have friends, and so do your muscles. For a moment, think of the muscular system as a party where people are looking for a date. You are the muscle, and you're looking for a bone. The tendon is your "wingman" (the one who makes the introductions to the opposite sex). A tendon helps muscles make contact with bones. There are tendons on each end of skeletal muscles because a muscle needs to be attached to two bones to make movement possible. Each muscle has *a point of origin* and a *point of insertion*. Muscles are attached to a stable bone at the point of origin and to a moving bone at the point of insertion, and this allows for movement when a muscle contracts and relaxes. And they all lived happily ever after.

Muscular expanding and contracting doesn't just happen in your biceps. It happens all over the body. Muscles support and maintain posture and produce body heat. They help form many internal organs and regulate the work those organs do behind the scenes (such as the heart, uterus, lungs, and intestines) even when the body is not moving. The muscles of arteries, intestines, heart, and stomach, for example, are always at work even when we aren't thinking of them. However, the silent work muscles do inside your body is wholly different from more obvious muscular work done by your arms and legs, for example.

Internal movement involves the contraction and relaxation of involuntary muscles, muscles that we cannot consciously control. For example, heartbeats are performed by cardiac muscles. Breathing and digestion are facilitated by muscles called *visceral* (involuntary) muscles, whereas external movement is accomplished by contraction and relaxation of muscles that are attached to bones. The muscles that provide this external movement are known as voluntary muscles, as they perform movements on command.

All bodily movement, whether lifting of an arm, or the beating of the heart, involves the contraction and relaxation of voluntary or involuntary muscles.

Classes of muscles

The class system is alive and well, at least as far as your muscles are concerned. There are three classes of muscles: skeletal, visceral, and cardiac.

  ✔ **Cardiac** (involuntary striated) muscle has branching fibers and forms most of the wall of the heart. Its contraction produces the heartbeat.

✔ **Skeletal** (voluntary *striated,* meaning striped) muscles, are attached to the skeleton. They are called voluntary, of course, because they are controlled by your will. This type of muscle can be easily seen by flexing the forearm, which makes the bicep muscle become hard and thick.

✔ **Visceral** (involuntary smooth) muscle is found in the stomach, intestines, and blood vessels, and cannot be controlled at will.

Unlike other muscle, cardiac (heart) muscle keeps beating even when removed from the body, as in a heart transplant. And even if it stops beating, it can be jump started with an external electrical charge Not so the other muscles.

Types of muscles

Oh, if it were only that easy. But there are also *types* of muscles. At first glance, the types of muscles are the same as the classes of muscle. But pay close attention and you'll see there are subtle differences. There are three *types* of muscles in the body.

Striated muscle

Striated muscles are also called skeletal or voluntary muscles. These are the muscles that move all the bones, as well as the face and the eyes. The body is able to consciously control the activity of a striated muscle.

Smooth muscle

The second type of muscle is *smooth muscle,* also known as visceral, involuntary or unstriated muscle. The body has no conscious control over smooth muscles, which move the internal organs such as the digestive tract. The smooth muscles are also found in blood vessels and secretory ducts leading from glands.

Skeletal muscle fibers are arranged in bundles, but smooth muscles form sheets of fibers that wrap around tubes and vessels.

Cardiac muscles

The third type of muscle is *cardiac muscle.* It is striated in appearance but is like smooth muscle in its actions. Movement of cardiac muscle cannot be consciously controlled. Cardiac muscle has branching fibers forming most of the wall of the heart and controlling the contractions producing the heartbeat.

Tell me more: Describing muscles

Oh sure, you could use good old, standard English adjectives to describe muscles and their characteristics, but why not have some fun? Try these descriptives on for size:

✔ **Gracilis:** Slender

✔ **Latissimus:** Wide

✔ **Longus:** Long

✔ **Orbicularis:** Surrounding

✔ **Rectus:** Straight

✔ **Serratus:** Sawtoothed

✔ **Transversus:** Crosswise

✔ **Vastus:** Great, big

Muscles and tendons

Now that you know the classes and types of muscles, let's take a more in-depth look at how they work. You already know that skeletal muscles, or striated muscles, are the muscles that move the bones of the body. Now get ready for the scoop on what makes it possible.

When a muscle *contracts*, one of the attached bones remains stationary, as a result of other muscles holding it in place. The point of attachment of the muscle to the stationary bone is called the *origin* or beginning of that muscle. When the muscle contracts, another bone to which it is attached, does move. The junction of the muscle to the bone that moves is called the *insertion* of the muscle. Near the point of insertion, the muscle narrows and is connected to the bone by a tendon. One type of tendon that helps attach bone to muscles is called an *aponeurosis*.

Round-up of the superficial muscles

Sometimes, being superficial isn't a bad thing. Take, for example, your *superficial* muscles, so named because these are the ones you're most likely to see with the naked eye. These workhorses of the muscular system help make you unique. Though they all have complicated-sounding names, they help your body perform everyday functions like picking up objects and smiling.

Figures 13-1 through 13-4 illustrate four major muscle groups.

> ✔ **Arm muscles** consist of the upper arm muscles, *biceps brachii* and *triceps brachii*. In the forearm (lower arm) are the *flexor* and *extensor muscles* of the hands and fingers.

✔ **Head and face muscles** include the *frontalis, temporalis, orbicularis oculi, orbicularis oris, occipitalis, mentalis, buccinator, zygomatic major* and *minor,* and the *masseter* muscle.

✔ **Shoulder and neck muscles** include the *sternocleidomastoid, pectoralis major, latissimus dorsi,* and *trapezius* muscle, leading to the *deltoid* muscle of the shoulder.

✔ **The major chest muscles** consist of the *diaphragm, pectoralis major,* the *rectus abdominis,* and the *external oblique.* Also associated with this region is the linea alba. The *linea alba* (meaning "white line") is a vertical band of connective muscular tissue that begins at the *xiphoid process* (sternum) and ends at the *symphysis pubis* (where hip bones meet).

✔ **The major muscles of the back** include the seventh cervical vertebra, infraspinatus, supraspinatus, latissimus dorsi, and the rhomboid major muscle.

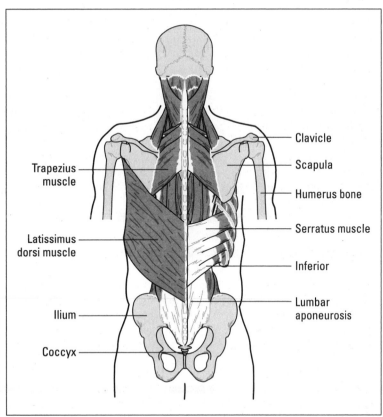

Figure 13-1:
Posterior
view of the
neck and
shoulder
muscles.

From LifeARTS®, Super Anatomy 1, ©2002, Lippincott Williams & Wilkins

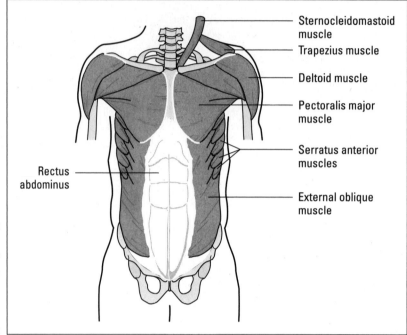

Figure 13-2:
Anterior
muscles
of the
chest and
abdomen.

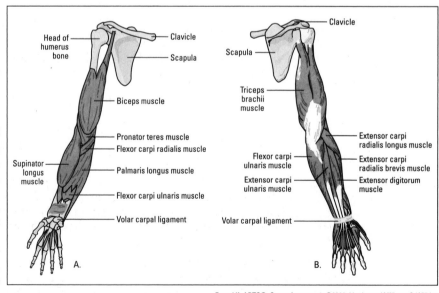

Figure 13-3:
The
muscles
of the
upper limb,
anterior
(A) and
posterior
(B).

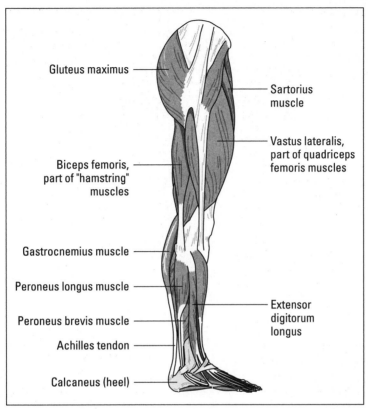

Gluteus maximus

Sartorius muscle

Vastus lateralis, part of quadriceps femoris muscles

Biceps femoris, part of "hamstring" muscles

Gastrocnemius muscle

Peroneus longus muscle

Peroneus brevis muscle

Extensor digitorum longus

Achilles tendon

Calcaneus (heel)

Figure 13-4: The muscles of the lower limb.

From LifeARTS®, Super Anatomy 1, ©2002, Lippincott Williams & Wilkins

The seventh cervical vertebra muscle is a muscle, whereas the seventh vertebra is a bone. Many muscles, tendons, and ligaments have the same name but don't have the same function. In this case, the 7th cervical muscle is a point of attachment aiding in support and movement of head and neck.

- ✔ **The pelvis and anterior thigh muscles** include the *tensor fascia lata,* the *adductors* of the thigh, the *vastus lateralis* and *vastus medialis*, the *rectus femoris*, and the *quadriceps*.

- ✔ **The lower leg muscles** from the knee to the ankle includes the *gastrocnemius,* which makes up a large portion of the calf muscles, the *tibialis anterior, soleus, peroneus longus*, and *peroneus brevis*. By the way, things aren't always what they seem: The *Achilles tendon* is technically classified as a muscle.

- ✔ **From the back, the buttocks** are composed of the *gluteus maximus* and *gluteus medius*. In the thigh, the *adductor magnus, vastus lateralis, gracilis*, whereas the *biceps femoris, semitendinosus* and *semimembranosus* combined comprise the hamstrings.

So, the moral of our muscle story is teamwork. Bones cannot move alone without being attached to muscle. Muscles cannot move alone, without being attached to stationary bones to allow support for that movement. Neither bones nor muscles could function without the attachments provided by the tendons and ligaments. Body movement then, is made possible by the bones and skeletal muscles working together in addition to the visceral and cardiac muscles that function to maintain the muscular rhythm of our vital organs. It's all one big, happy family of muscles.

Muscular Roots and Suffixes

Let's put your new-found expertise into practice by breaking down the root words into meanings and useful applications. The roots are essential medical terminology knowledge, because once you master these roots (good ol' Greek and Latin ones, that is), you can break down any muscular-related word and discover its meaning.

Don't confuse *myo* (muscle) with *myelo* (bone marrow).

Root words, combining forms, and suffixes associated with the skeletal system include the ones shown in Tables 13-1 and 13-2.

Table 13-1	Breaking Down Your Muscular Roots
Root Word	*What It Means*
Duct/o	To draw
Fasci/o	Fascia (band of tissue surrounding muscle)
Flex/o	Bend
Leiomy/o	Smooth visceral muscle
My/o	Muscle
Myocardi/o	Heart muscle
Myos/o	Muscle
Pronati/o	Facing down or backward
Rhabdomy/o	Skeletal or striated muscle
Sarc/o	Soft, fleshy, or connective tissue
Supinati/o	Facing up or forward
Tens/o	Stretch

Unofficialoma

Unofficial but not uncommon slang includes *incidentaloma*, which refers to something found on a study, which is not particularly important or else not relevant to the study at hand, but still worth noting. There's also *fascinoma*, something weird and noteworthy: "Hey, check this out, it's a real fascinoma."

Table 13-2	Muscular Suffixes
Suffix	*What It Means*
-algia	Pain in fibrous tissue
-desis	Surgical fixation
-ectomy	Surgical removal or excision
-gram	Record
-graphy	The process of recording
-itis	Inflammation
-ology	Study of
-oma	Tumor or mass
-otomy	To cut into
-pathy	Disease
-rrhaphy	Suture repair

Action Item: The Movement of Your Muscles

Your muscles do a serious amount of work every single hour of every day. Though you may be reading this book propped up on some pillows while munching corn chips, your muscles are at work — muscles are moving your eyes across the words so you can read and comprehend, smooth muscles are working your organs, and superficial muscles are helping keep your body upright. Turns out, for every muscular action, luckily for you, there is a word to describe it. Here are just a few muscular action words to remember:

- **Abduction:** Movement of drawing away from the center of the body (such as fingers spread apart)

- **Adduction:** Movement of drawing toward the middle of the body (i.e. fingers held together)

- **Eversion:** Turning outward

- **Extension:** Movement in which a limb is placed in a straight position

- **Flexion:** Movement in which a limb is bent

- **Inversion:** Turning inward

- **Pronation:** Movement that turns the palm of the hand downward

- **Rotation:** Turning around on its own axis

- **Supination:** Movement that turns the palm of the hand upward

To remember the difference between *-ectomy* and *-otomy*, remember *-ectomy* with *e for exit or excision* and *-otomy* for *o to open only*.

Common Muscular Conditions

Muscular conditions are fairly common in people of all ages and backgrounds. From tennis elbow to the enigmatic fibromyalgia, the muscular system can take a real beating. Here are the most common muscular conditions:

- **Bursitis:** Inflammation of the bursa sac, which lines the joint and provides smooth joint movement

- **Fibromyalgia:** Pain in fibrous tissues of muscles, tendons, or ligaments

- **Myoparalysis:** Paralysis of a muscle

- **Tennis elbow:** The tendon that connects the arm muscle to elbow becomes inflamed due to the repetitive use of the arm

  The actual medical term for this is *lateral* or *medial epicondylitis* (*lateral* if referring to the bump on the outside of the elbow, *medial* to the bump on the inside).

- **Tendinitis or tendonitis:** Inflammation of a tendon

- **Tenosynovitis:** Inflammation of the tendon and the sheath around it, often in a finger or the wrist

Finding the Culprit: Muscular Diseases and Pathology

Some of the most serious diseases affect the muscular system. From diseases that affect facial movement to the full-body atrophy of Lou Gehrig's disease, these diseases are all challenging:

- **Amyotrophic lateral sclerosis (ALS):** Movement disorder or muscle atrophy with degeneration of nerves in the spinal cord and lower region of the brain, also known as Lou Gehrig's disease

- **Dupuytren's contracture:** Disease affecting the *palmar fascia* of the hand, causing the ring finger and little finger to contract towards the palm

- **Leiomyoma:** Benign tumor of smooth muscle

- **Leiomyosarcoma:** Malignant tumor of smooth muscle

- **Myasthenia gravis:** Lack of muscle strength with paralysis, characterized by weakness of muscles of the face and jaw, with difficulty swallowing

- **Myosarcoma:** Malignant tumor of muscle tissue

- **Muscular dystrophy:** Inherited disease characterized by progressive weakness and degeneration of muscle fibers without involvement of the nervous system

- **Polymyalgia rheumatica:** Muscle pain, common in shoulder or pelvis, without arthritis or signs of muscle distress

- **Rotator cuff disease:** Inflammation of tendons, and if they fuse you have a larger problem, a condition called *frozen shoulder* or *adhesive capsulitis*

- **Torticollis:** Acute myositis of the cervical muscles (wryneck)

Testing, Testing: Muscular Radiology and Diagnostic tests

Though the list of muscular conditions and diseases is quite long, there are some simple diagnostic tests doctors can perform to diagnose most muscular ailments.

> ✔ **Electromyogram (EMG)** is a record of electric activity in a muscle. This procedure is done to diagnose carpal tunnel syndrome. *Electromyography* is an electrical recording of activity in a muscle.

> ✔ **MRI (magnetic resonance imaging):** The gold standard for making pictures of soft tissue such as fascia, tendons, ligaments and muscle.

> ✔ **X-ray:** Picture of the bones.

Paging Dr. Terminology: Muscular Surgeries and Procedures

Now that your muscles have been poked, prodded, tested, and diagnosed, it's time to fix what's broken. Most of these procedures are surgical in nature.

Many surgeries are performed arthroscopically, through a scope inserted into or near a joint space, with one lone endoscopic rogue, *Palmar uniportal endoscopic carpal tunnel release*. This is also called a *Mirza technique*, an endoscopic method for release of carpal tunnel, previously accomplished by open surgery.

The surgical players are

> ✔ **Fasciectomy:** Excision of fascia (fibrous band or membrane of tissue surrounding muscle)

> ✔ **Myoplasty:** Surgical repair of a muscle

> ✔ **Myorrhaphy:** Suturing of a muscle

> ✔ **Tenodesis:** Surgical fixation of a tendon

> ✔ **Tenomyoplasty:** Surgical repair of a tendon and muscle

> ✔ **Tenorrhaphy:** Suturing of a tendon

> ✔ **Tenotomy:** Incision of a tendon

It's All Related: More Muscular Terms

While the makeup of the muscular system is pretty straightforward, there are still all sorts of useful terms you need to know in order to communicate about your muscles. Try a few of the words from Table 13-3 on for size.

Table 13-3	Common Muscular Vocabulary
Word	*What It Means*
Articulation	Joint
Atrophy	Without development, wasting away of a muscle
Bradykinesia	Slow body movement
Diathermy	Heat applied to deep tissues
Dyskinesia	Difficult body movement
Dystrophy	Abnormal development
Fascia	Band of tissue surrounding muscle
Fasciitis	Inflammation of fascia
Hyperkinesia	Excessive body movement or overactivity
Kinesiology	The study of movement
Ligament	Binds bone to bone
Myasthenia	Muscle weakness
Myalgia	Muscle pain
Myology	The study of muscles
Myoclonus	Muscle relaxation and contraction in rapid succession
Myopathy	Any muscular disease
Tendon	Connective tissue binding muscles to bones
Tenodynia	Pain in a tendon
Tenosynovitis	Inflammation of the tendon and synovial membrane

Chapter 14

Skin Deep: Skin, Glands, Nails, and Hair

In This Chapter

▶ Finding out how your integumentary system works

▶ Determining root words, prefixes, and suffixes appropriate to this system

▶ Using terminology of the integumentary system to discuss common conditions and diseases

▶ Discovering the right terms to use when diagnosing problems

*Y*our skin (the body's largest organ), glands, nails, and hair — also known as the *integumentary* system — serve as the "public face" of your body. Consider it your marketing team, letting the world know by their condition how healthy the rest of your body is. Healthy skin, along with accessory organs glands, hair, and nails, are the hallmarks of healthy insides, so care for them accordingly.

Layers of Skin

Like an onion, your skin has several layers, and there is much more to it than what you see with the naked eye. The skin is a system of specialized tissue, containing glands that secrete fluids, nerves that carry impulses, and blood vessels that assist in the regulation of body temperature.

Integumentum means "covering." This system is the body's covering, made up mostly of skin, but with the help of the accessory organs.

The skin has almost as many jobs as it has layers. The skin acts as a protective membrane that is a barrier against microorganisms, and it protects organs from injury. Skin helps maintain and regulate body temperature and acts as a receptor for sensation (hot, cold, touch, and pain). The skin helps rid the body of waste products. It also guards deeper tissues of the body against excessive loss of water, salts, and heat. Secretions from the skin are somewhat acidic in nature and contribute to its ability to fight off bacterial invasion.

The skin has the large responsibility of keeping you cool. The many different tissues in the skin help maintain the body temperature. Nerve fibers coordinate this *thermoregulation* by carrying messages to the skin from heat centers in the brain that are sensitive to changes in the body temperature. Nerve impulses cause blood vessels to dilate to bring blood to the surface where the heat can dissipate and cause sweat glands to produce the watery secretion that evaporates, thereby acting as your cooling system.

The skin is the most important player in the integumentary system, and is made up of three layers. The outer layer is the epidermis, a thin, cellular membrane layer. The second layer is the dermis, dense fibrous connective tissue. The third layer is the subcutaneous tissue, fat-containing tissue that joins the skin to underlying muscle.

The structure of skin varies throughout the body. It is stretchable and tough and has different thicknesses. It is thick on the palms of the hands and soles of the feet, but thin on the eyelids. The skin is initially firm and elastic, but with age, becomes wrinkled, drier, and saggy, especially around the eyes, mouth, and neck. The skin covering palms of the hand and soles of the feet is different from that covering the rest of the body. The skin on fingers and toes has patterns of ridges that never change and are unique for each individual, and, as you know from crime dramas, provide a basis for the use of fingerprints as a means of positive identification.

Epidermis

The *epidermis* is the outer, totally cellular layer of skin. It is composed of epithelium. *Epithelium* covers both internal and external surfaces of the body. The epidermis has no blood vessels, lymphatic vessels, connective tissue, cartilage, or fat. It depends on the deeper dermis, or corium, layer and its network of capillaries for nourishment. Oxygen and nutrients from the capillaries in the dermis pass through tissue fluid, supplying nourishment to the deeper levels of the epidermis.

The deepest layer of the epidermis is called the *basal layer.* Cells in the basal layer are always growing and multiplying. As the basal layer cells divide, they are pushed upwards and away from the blood supply of the dermis layer by a steady stream of younger cells. These cells shrink, lose their nuclei, die, and become filled with a hard protein called *keratin*. They are then called *horny cells*, reflecting their composition of keratin. Within a 3–4 week period after living as a basal cell in the deepest part of the epidermis, the horny keratinized cell is sloughed off from the surface of the skin. The epidermis, then, is constantly renewing itself.

Cells die at the same rate at which they are born. The basal layer of the epidermis contains cells called melanocytes. *Melanocytes* contain a black pigment called *melanin*. The amount of melanin accounts for the color differences in skin. Darker skin possesses more active melanocytes, not a greater number of melanocytes. Melanin in the epidermis is vital for protection against harmful ultraviolet radiation, which can manifest as skin cancers.

Individuals, who through a flaw in their chemical make-up are incapable of forming melanin, are called *albino*, meaning white. Their skin and hair are white and their eyes are red (because of the absence of pigment, the tiny blood vessels are visible in the iris).

Dermis

The *dermis*, the second layer, below the epidermis, is also called the *corium*. The dermis differs from the epidermis in that it is living tissue composed of blood, lymph vessels, and nerve fibers, as well as the accessory organs of the skin. These accessories include the hair follicles, sweat glands, and oil glands.

To support this system of nerves, vessels, and glands, the dermis contains connective tissue cells and fibers. The dermis is composed of different types of connective tissue cells: fibroblasts, histiocytes, and mast cells. *Fibroblast* cells act to repair an injury to the skin. *Histiocytes* protect the body by surrounding foreign materials. *Mast cells* contain histamine, a substance released in allergies that causes itching.

Fibers in the dermis are composed of collagen. *Collagen*, meaning "glue," is a fibrous protein material found in bone, cartilage, tendons, and ligaments as well as the skin. It is tough, but also flexible. In an infant, collagen is loose and delicate but it becomes harder as the body ages. Collagen fibers support and protect the blood and nerve networks that pass through the dermis.

Hair shafts in the dermis have bundles of involuntary muscle called *arrector pili* attached to hair follicles. When you are frightened or cold, these muscles contract, the hair stands up, and "goosebumps" appear on the skin.

Subcutaneous layer

The subcutaneous layer of the skin is made up of connective tissue that specializes in the formation of fat. *Lipocytes*, plentiful in the subcutaneous layer, manufacture and store large amounts of fat. Areas of the body vary as far as fat deposition is concerned. This layer of skin is important in protecting deeper tissues of the body and also acts as a heat insulator. The subcutaneous layer connects the dermis to the muscles and organs below it. Its fat tissue insulates inner structures from temperature extremes.

Glands, Both Sebaceous and Sudoriferous

The skin has two types of glands that, as accessory organs, produce important secretions. These glands under the skin's surface are called the sebaceous (oil) glands and the sudoriferous (sweat) glands.

The *sebaceous* glands produce an oily secretion called *sebum*, whereas the *sudoriferous* glands produce a watery secretion called *sweat*. Sebum and sweat are carried to the outer edges of the skin by ducts and excreted through openings in the skin called *pores*. Sebum helps lubricate the skin. Sebaceous glands are closely associated with hair follicles, and their ducts open into the hair follicle through which the sebum is released.

Sebaceous glands are influenced by sex hormones. This causes them to be overactive at puberty and underactive in old age. This explains the excess oil production of the skin at puberty and gradual drying of the skin as we age.

Stinking it up: Your sweat glands

Sweat gets a bad rap for being smelly when, in fact, it's not your fault. Your body's smell is caused by bacteria. Sweat or perspiration is almost pure water, with dissolved materials such as salt making up less than 1 percent of its total composition. Sweat is actually colorless and odorless. The odor produced when sweat accumulates is due to the action of bacteria on it.

Certain sweat glands, active only from puberty onward and larger than ordinary sweat glands, are concentrated near the reproductive organs and in the *axillae* (armpits). These glands secrete an odorless sweat that contains substances that are easily broken down by skin bacteria. The breakdown products are responsible for the characteristic "human body odor." So the next time someone tells you your sweat stinks, you can say, "I beg to differ. My bacteria is the culprit."

The *ceruminous glands* are classified as modified sweat glands and are found in the ear canal. These glands produce a yellow waxy substance called *cerumen* (ear wax).

Sudoriferous (sweat) glands are tiny coiled glands found on almost all body surfaces. You have about 2 million of them in your body. There are many more in the palms of the hands, and you'd fine approximately 3000 glands per square inch on the sole of your foot. The tiny openings on the surface are called *pores*. Sweat helps cool the body as it evaporates from the skin surface. Nerve fibers under the skin detect pain, temperature, pressure, and touch. The adjustment of the body to its environment depends on the sensory messages relayed to the brain and spinal cord by the sensitive nerve endings in the skin.

Diaphoresis comes from the Greek *dia,* meaning "through," and *phoreo* meaning "I carry." Translated, it means "the carrying through of perspiration."

Figure 14-1 illustrates the layers of the skin and some of its structures.

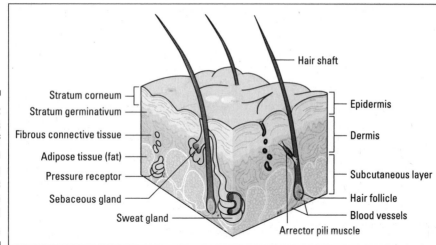

Figure 14-1: Cross section of the skin showing layers and some specialized structures.

From LifeARTS®, Super Anatomy 1, ©2002, Lippincott Williams & Wilkins

Hair and Nails

A *hair fiber* is composed of a network of horny cells (hold your giggles, please) filled with hard protein called *keratin*. Hair growth is similar to the growth of the epidermal layer of the skin. Deep-lying cells in hair roots move forward through the hair *follicles,* or shafts, that hold the hair fiber. *Melanocytes* located at the root of hair follicles supply the melanin pigment for the hair fiber. Hair color depends on the amount of melanin present, as it does with the color of the skin. Because hormone production decreases as we get older, the hair loses color and becomes transparent (which we see as gray).

Nails are hard keratin plates that cover the *dorsal* (top) surface of the last bone of each toe and finger. Nails are composed of horny cells that are cemented together and can extend indefinitely until cut or broken. A nail grows in thickness and length by division of the cells of the nerve root, at the base of the nail plate. Nails grow approximately 1 millimeter a week, which means that fingernails may regrow completely in 3–5 months. Toenails grow more slowly than fingernails, but if you have lost a toenail due to a nasty stubbing incident, it will come back eventually.

Integumentary Root Words

Now that you've gotten to know the specific parts of the integumentary system a bit better, it's time to put your expertise into practice by tracking down the meaning of root words and checking out their useful applications. The roots are essential medical terminology knowledge, because once you master these roots (good ol' Greek and Latin ones, that is), you can break down any hair/skin/nail/gland-related word and discover its meaning. Table 14-1 lists integumentary root words.

Table 14-1	Breaking Down Your Integumentary Roots
Root Word	*What It Means*
Aden/o	Gland
Adip/o	Fat
Albin/o	White
Aut/o	Self
Bi/o	Life
Blephar/o	Eyelid
Carcin/o	Carcinoma (cancer)
Cutane/o	Skin
Cry/o	Cold
Cyan/o	Blue
Derm/o, Dermat/o	Skin
Diaphor/o	Profuse sweating
Erythem/o	Red
Hidr/o	Sweat
Histi/o	Tissue
Kerat/o	Hard, horny

Root Word	What It Means
Leuk/o	White
Lip/o	Fat
Melan/o	Black
Myc/o	Fungus
Necr/o	Death (cell or body)
Onych/o	Nail
Papill/o	Nipple-like
Pil/o	Hair
Py/o	Pus
Rhytid/o	Wrinkle
Sclera/o	Hardening
Seb/o	Sebum
Squam/o	Scale
Steat/o	Fat, sebum
Trich/o	Hair
Xer/o	Dry
Xanth/o	Yellow

Herpes comes from the Greek word *herpo* meaning "to creep along." It is descriptive of the course and type of skin lesion.

Table 14-2 lists prefixes and suffixes pertaining to your hair, nails, skin, and glands.

Table 14-2	Common Integumentary Prefixes and Suffixes
Prefix	**What It Means**
Epi-	On, over, upon
Para-	Beside, beyond, around
Per	Through
Sub-	Under, below
Suffix	**What It Means**
-itis	Inflammation
-malacia	Softening

(continued)

Table 14-2 *(continued)*

Prefix	What It Means
-opsy	View of, viewing
-orrhea	Flow, excessive discharge
-phagia	Eating or swallowing
-plasty	Surgical repair

Common Integumentary Conditions

Of all the conditions that plague the integumentary system, ones affecting the skin tend to be the most obvious and troublesome issues. From that odd, discolored freckle on your arm to run-of-the-mill acne, the list of unsavory and often embarrassing lesions is long. Take a look:

- **Bulla:** Large vesicle or blister (plural: *bullae*)
- **Comedo:** Common blackhead caused by a buildup of sebum and keratin in a skin pore (plural: *comedones*)
- **Cyst:** Small sac or pouch containing fluid or semisolid fluid
- **Fissure:** Groove or crack-like sore
- **Macule:** A discolored lesion that lies flush with the skin (freckles, tattoo marks, and moles)
- **Papule:** Solid elevation of the skin
- **Polyp:** Mushroom-like growth extending on a stalk
- **Pustule:** Discrete raised area of pus on the skin
- **Ulcer:** Open sore or erosion of the skin
- **Vesicle:** Collection of clear fluid (blister)
- **Wheal:** Smooth elevated area that is red and itchy (such as *hives*).

Lesions aren't alone, though. A host of conditions affect the entire integumentary system. The majority of them, however, still affect the skin more than other parts of the system:

- **Alopecia:** Hair loss. Can result normally from aging process or be drug or illness-induced
- **Cicatrix:** Scar left by a healed wound

✔ **Ecchymosis:** Purplish macular bruise, hemorrhage into the skin

✔ **Keloid:** Abnormally raised, thickened scar

✔ **Petechia:** Small pinpoint hemorrhage (plural: *petechiae*)

✔ **Pruritus:** Itching, associated with forms of *dermatitis*

✔ **Purpura:** Merging ecchymoses with petechiae

✔ **Urticaria:** Hives with localized swelling with itching

✔ **Vitiligo:** Loss of pigment in area of skin or milk-white patch

Another important one is *burn*: injury to tissues caused by heat, flame, electricity, chemicals, or radiation contact. A *first-degree burn* is superficial with no blister and superficial damage in epidermis. A *second-degree burn,* or *partial thickness burn*, blisters and causes damage to epidermis and dermis. A *third-degree burn* is full-thickness, damaging the epidermis, dermis, and subcutaneous layer.

Finding the Culprit: Integumentary Diseases and Pathology

Once again, the skin is the major player when it comes to ailments. Surely the hair, nails, and glands won't feel too left out of this motley group of pathological conditions and diseases. The most popular pathological conditions include the following:

✔ **Acne:** Inflammatory pustular eruption of skin (*acne vulgaris* is the common variety)

✔ **Decubitus ulcer:** Bedsore

✔ **Eczema:** Inflammatory skin disease with reddened papular lesion; a common allergic reaction in children

✔ **Gangrene:** Death of tissue associated with loss of blood supply

✔ **Impetigo:** Bacterial inflammatory skin disease presenting with vesicles, pustules, and crusted lesions; caused by bacteria

✔ **Psoriasis:** Chronic (ongoing) skin ailment with silver-gray scales covering red patches

✔ **Scleroderma:** Disorder affecting all connective tissue that causes abnormal tissue thickening usually on fingers, hands or face

✔ **Tinea:** Infection of the skin caused by a fungus

There are also viral diseases that result in eruptions of skin from the infection. These include

- ✔ **Rubella:** German measles
- ✔ **Rubeola:** Measles
- ✔ **Varicella:** Chickenpox

Sometimes, the skin experiences skin *neoplasms*, also known as "new growth." These are often benign and can include the following:

- ✔ **Hemangioma:** A cluster of blood vessels that make an abnormal but benign growth, often protruding from the skin; some birthmarks are hemangiomas
- ✔ **Keratosis:** Thickened area of the epidermis (wart, callus)
- ✔ **Nevus:** Mole (plural: *nevi*)
- ✔ **Seborrheic keratosis:** Thick, flattened, beige/brown plaques that appear commonly on hands and face with age; sometimes called senile warts
- ✔ **Verruca:** Warts

Unfortunately, the news from the dermatologist can often be serious enough to warrant further testing and may involve the "Big C" — cancer. *Basal cell carcinoma*, for example, is a malignant tumor of the basal cell layer of epidermis. It is the most common type of skin cancer and is slow growing, usually occurring on upper half of the face near the nose. It does not spread. *Squamous cell carcinoma* is a malignant tumor of the *squamous epithelial* cells of the epidermis. This tumor may arise from actinic or sun-related keratoses and may metastasize to lymph nodes. *Malignant melanoma* is a cancerous tumor composed of melanocytes. Tumors often metastasize or spread to liver, lung, and brain. Finally, *mycoses fungoides* is a rare chronic skin disease caused by the infiltration of malignant *lymphocytes*. It is characterized by large red raised areas that spread and ulcerate; malignant cells may involve lymph nodes.

Testing, Testing: Integumentary Radiology and Diagnostic tests

There are two major ways that dermatologists and their colleagues diagnose issues with the integumentary system by taking a tissue sample from the body. These two types of tests involve the winning combination of bacteria and fungus. Bacterial analysis and fungal testing are laboratory tests in which the doctor takes cultures or swabs and then examines them in the lab.

✓ **Bacterial analysis** is performed by taking a sample of a purulent or pus-filled material or exudates (fluid that accumulates in the space or passes out of tissue). The sample is then sent for examination to determine what type of bacteria is present.

✓ **Fungal testing** occurs when scrapings from skin lesion are placed on a growth medium for several weeks and then examined for evidence of fungal growth.

Paging Dr. Terminology: Integumentary Surgeries and Procedures

Many of the more common, everyday integumentary conditions can be fixed or improved via in-office or outpatient procedures. These procedures aren't necessarily pretty, but they sure do get the job done. They are as follows:

✓ **Debridement** is the removal of dirt, foreign material, or damaged tissue from a wound to prevent infection and promote healing.

✓ **Incision and drainage** involve cutting open a lesion such as an abscess to remove or drain contents.

✓ **Intradermal test** is performed by injection of a reactive substance between layers of the skin to observe for a reaction. This test is used to detect sensitivity to infectious agents such as *tuberculosis* (the Mantoux test) or PPD (purified protein derivative) test, or the test for diphtheria (the Schick test). Strong reactions indicate ongoing infection, or previous exposure.

✓ **Patch skin test** is performed by applying a piece of gauze or paper to the skin, on which has been placed an allergy-causing substance. If area becomes red and swollen, the result is positive.

✓ **Punch biopsy** is used to obtain tissue in cases in which complete excision is not necessary or possible. Involves using a surgical instrument that removes a core of tissue by rotation of its sharp edge.

✓ **Sclerotherapy** is used in the treatment of varicose veins. Injecting the vein with a *sclerosing solution* irritates the tissue, causes swelling, and closes off the vein.

✓ **Skin biopsy** is removal of living tissue for microscopic examination. Skin lesions that might be in danger of producing a malignant change are removed and sent for pathologic examination.

✓ **Skin scratch test** involves making several scratches in the skin and injecting a very minimal amount of test material into the scratches; a test is considered negative if no reaction occurs.

We Americans are a vain people, no doubt. Cosmetic surgery is practically a pastime in the United States. But consider that this type of surgical procedure can be about more than looking and feeling younger. Cosmetic surgery is a vital field that helps people recover from all sorts of serious wounds. For example, cosmetic surgery helps the person with the scarred face caused in an auto accident, the woman mourning the loss of a breast to cancer, or the child born with a facial deformity. Some of the most common surgical procedures in this field are the following:

- **Blepharoplasty** is surgical reduction of the upper and lower eyelids.

- **Cryotherapy** involves destruction of tissue by freezing with liquid nitrogen.

- **Dermabrasion** means scraping away of the top layer of skin using sandpaper or wire brushes to remove tattoos or disfigured skin.

- **Dermatoplasty** is surgical reconstruction of the skin. Typically, the surgical replacement of injured or diseased skin.

- **Electrolysis** is destruction of tissue by electricity and is used to remove unwanted body hair.

- **Laser therapy** involves removal of skin lesions such as *papillomas* and *hemangiomas* using an intense beam of light. This can also be used to remove tattoos or warts from around the nails or on the soles of feet.

- **Liposuction** is surgical removal of fat from subcutaneous tissue by means of suction.

- **Rhytidectomy** means removal of wrinkles by removal of excess facial skin. Also known as a facelift.

It's All Related: More Integumentary Terms

The integumentary system involves many different components that are not necessarily outwardly similar, from skin and hair to nails and glands. As such, there are tons of vocabulary words for this system. Table 14-3 shows a sampling.

Table 14-3	Common Integumentary Vocabulary
Word	*What It Means*
Abrasion	Scraping away of superficial layer of injured skin
Adenoma	Glandular tumor
Albinism	Lack of pigment in skin, hair, and eyes
Albino	Person with skin deficient in pigment or melanin
Adipose	Pertaining to fat
Anhidrosis	Lack of sweat
Collagen	Structural protein found in skin and connective tissues
Cuticle	Band of epidermis extending from nail wall to nail surface
Dermatitis	Inflammation of the skin
Dermatology	Study of the skin and its diseases
Dermatologist	Physician who specializes in skin and its diseases
Diaphoresis	Profuse sweating
Epithelium	Layer of skin forming the outer and inner surfaces of body
Erythema	Red discoloration of the skin
Histiotoma	Fatty tumor of sebaceous gland
Hypodermic	Under the skin
Hyperhidrosis	Excessive secretion of sweat
Hyperkeratosis	Excessive growth of the outer layer of skin
Keratin	Hard protein material found in epidermis, hair and nails
Lipocyte	Fat cell
Lipoma	Tissue or mass containing fat
Lunula	The half-moon shaped white area at base of the nail
Melanin	Black pigment formed by melanocytes
Onychomycosis	Fungal infection of nail
Seborrhea	Increased discharge of sebum from glands

Chapter 15

It Depends on Your Perception: The Sensory Systems

In This Chapter

▶ Seeing how your sensory system works

▶ Ferreting out root words, prefixes, and suffixes appropriate to this system

▶ Using terminology of the sensory system to discuss common conditions and diseases

▶ Sensing the right terms to use when diagnosing problems

*Y*ou can thank your sensory systems for all the fun you get to have in life. While your other, also very important, systems handle the background work that keeps you running, the senses let your body have a little fun. What you see, hear, smell, touch, and taste makes life the enjoyable experience it is. So the next time you're smelling some truly fantastic barbecue or watching a dazzling fireworks display, be grateful for your senses.

The Eye

For humans, the eye is the most important sense organ — the Big Kahuna of the senses. Sight provides the most information for us, for what we see, of course, but that includes what we can read. The eye is located in the *orbit* (the bony protective cavity of the skull). The eye lets light in, focuses it, transforms it into nerve impulses, and sends these impulses to the brain.

Here's how: Light rays enter the eye via an adjustable opening, the dark center of the eye, called the *pupil*, which regulates the amount of light allowed in. Behind the pupil is the *lens*, which focuses the light. The lens is not rigid and it can adjust its shape in order to adapt to near and far objects.

The light is focused by the lens into the back of the eye, where it strikes the *retina*. The retina transforms the focused image into nerve impulses that travel along the optic nerve to the *occipital lobe* of the brain for processing.

Figure 15-1 gives you a peek inside the eye.

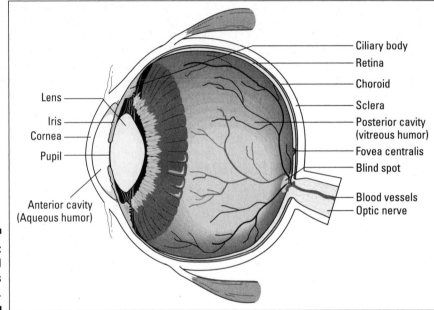

Ciliary body
Retina
Choroid
Sclera
Posterior cavity (vitreous humor)
Fovea centralis
Blind spot
Blood vessels
Optic nerve

Lens
Iris
Cornea
Pupil
Anterior cavity (Aqueous humor)

Figure 15-1: Internal structures of the eye.

From LifeARTS®, Super Anatomy 1, ©2002, Lippincott Williams & Wilkins

The eye consists of the *inner eye* (the eyeball) and the *outer eye* (the facial structures and eye muscles surrounding the eye).

Eye like it short

Here are some common abbreviations for the eye. You might hear these in conversation or see them on medical charts.

✔ **OD:** Right eye (oculus dexter)

✔ **OS:** Left eye (oculus sinister)

✔ **OU:** Each eye (oculus uterque)

✔ **PERRLA:** Pupils equal, round, and reactive to light and accommodation

✔ **VA:** Visual acuity

✔ **VF:** Visual field

Check your lenses

The lens is not considered part of one of the layers of the eye. As light passes through, it is bent. The bending is called *refraction*. The refracted light must be focused on the retina for a clear image. In order to focus light, the lens changes shape. The ciliary muscles change its shape to allow for clear vision of far and near objects. This lens changing is called *accommodation*. When a person reaches his or her 40s, the lens loses some of its elasticity, causing difficulty focusing light from near objects. Reading glasses provide the refraction that the lens can no longer perform. The lens loses its transparent quality with age, becoming thick and dense and sometimes opaque and cloudy and interfering with the refraction of light rays. This results in a common condition, cataracts. Cataracts, once a leading cause of serious vision lost, are now routinely removed surgically.

Inner eye

The inner eye is made up of three layers.

The outer layer contains the cornea and the sclera. The *cornea* is the transparent anterior portion of the eye. It allows light in and aids in the focusing of light onto the back of the eye. The *sclera* is the white of the eye, providing a protective covering for the eyeball.

The middle layer, the *uvea*, consists of the choroids, the ciliary body, and the iris. The *choroids*, the inner lining of the sclera, contain blood vessels that nourish the eye. The *ciliary body* consists of the ciliary muscles and the ciliary process. The muscles adjust the shape of the lens for focusing, and the process produces a watery substance, *aqueous humor*, bathing the anterior region of the eye. The *iris* is the circular colored portion of the eye. The opening in the iris, the pupil, regulates the amount of light that enters the eye. In bright light, muscle fibers in the iris contract the pupil. These muscles relax in dimmer light, and the pupil resumes its normal size. Radial muscles in the iris enlarge the pupil beyond normal size when a person is stressed or excited, called *dilation*.

The inner layer is the *retina*, which has layers of nervous tissue called *cones* and *rods*. Each of your eyes has approximately 6 million cones and 120 million rods in the retina. The cones are more sensitive in light than the rods. Color and sharpness of vision depend on the cone cells. Rods function better in dim light and are helpful in night vision. One small area of the retina has no cones or rods and doesn't produce a visual image. Called the *optic disc* or *blind spot*, it's the entry point for the major blood vessels of the eye and where the optic nerve crosses from the brain into the eye.

In front of and in back of the lens are two cavities. The *anterior (front) cavity* contains *aqueous humor* produced by the ciliary processes. This watery fluid flows freely from the posterior chamber, through the pupil, to the anterior chamber. Inability to drain aqueous humor causes increased *intraocular pressure*. This condition, known as *glaucoma*, can result in blindness because of damage caused to the retina and optic nerve, by the extra pressure. Equal production and drainage maintains the equilibrium of the intraocular pressure. The *posterior (back) cavity* of the eye is filled with clear, jelly-like material called *vitreous humor*. This preserves the spherical shape of the eyeball, holding the retina firmly against the choroid. Both the aqueous and vitreous humors function to further refract light rays.

Outer eye

The outer eye consists of the orbital cavity, the ocular muscles, the eyelids, conjunctival membrane, and lacrimal apparatus. The *orbital cavity* is the bony depression that the eyeball fits. *Ocular muscles* attach to the sclera and move the eye. *Eyelids* shield the eye from light, dust, and trauma. The *conjunctival membrane* lining the eyelids and the anterior part of the eye exposed to the air provides protection and lubrication.

The *lacrimal apparatus* produces, delivers, and drains tears from the eye, providing cleaning and lubricating. The *lacrimal glands* produce the tears, which are continuously delivered to the eyes by the *lacrimal ducts*. Small openings called *punctae* drain tears from the eyes into channels in the nose. This is the reason you nose runs when you cry. Tears clean and lubricate the eye as well as fight infectious microorganisms.

Cataract comes from the Greek *kato,* meaning "down," and *raktos,* meaning "precipice." Combined, they can be interpreted as "waterfall." Through a cataract, sight is like a waterfall or misty. *Glaucoma* — Greek *glaukos* — means "blue-grey," and *oma* means "a condition." In glaucoma, a gray color replaces the black pupil.

The Ear

The ear has two functions: to hear and to help provide the body's balance or equilibrium. We can hear because sound waves vibrate through the ear where they are transformed into nerve impulses that are then carried to the brain. The sensations of sound are heard within the nerve fibers of the cerebral cortex.

Figure 15-2 shows the different parts of the ear.

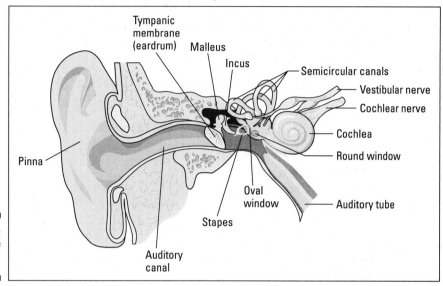

Tympanic membrane (eardrum)
Malleus
Incus
Semicircular canals
Vestibular nerve
Cochlear nerve
Cochlea
Round window
Pinna
Oval window
Auditory tube
Stapes
Figure 15-2:
Anatomy of the ear.
Auditory canal

From LifeARTS®, Super Anatomy 1, ©2002, Lippincott Williams & Wilkins

The ear is divided into three separate regions: the outer, middle, and inner ear. The outer and middle ears look after the conduction of sound waves through the ear. The inner ear contains the structures that carry the waves to the brain.

The short version of your ears

Some of the most common ear-related abbreviations include

- **AC:** Air conduction
- **AD:** Right ear (auris dextra)
- **AS:** Left ear (auris sinistra)
- **AU:** Both ears (aures unitas)

- **BC:** Bone conduction
- **HD:** Hearing distance
- **ENT:** Ear, nose, and throat
- **OM:** Otitis media

Outer ear

Sound waves are encouraged toward the ear canal by the *auricle*, or *pinna*, the visible outer ear, the hard, arching cartilage that forms the outer ear curve, the *tragus*, that hard little flap of cartilage that sticks out in front of the ear canal, and the earlobe.

From the pinna, the *external auditory meatus* is lined with numerous glands that secrete a yellowish waxy substance called *cerumen*. Cerumen (ear wax) lubricates and protects the ear. Sound waves travel through the auditory canal and strike the *tympanic membrane* or *eardrum*, located between the outer and middle ear.

Middle ear

As the eardrum vibrates, it moves three small bones or *ossicles* that make up the middle ear. Ossicles conduct the sound waves through the middle ear. These bones in the order of their vibration are the *malleus*, the *incus,* and the *stapes*. As the stapes moves, it touches a membrane called the *oval window*, which separates the middle ear from the inner ear. Another part of the middle ear is the *auditory* or *eustachian tube*, a canal leading from the middle ear to the pharynx. The eustachian tube equalizes air pressure on both sides of the eardrum.

Inner ear

The inner ear is also called the *labyrinth* because of its circular, maze-like structure. The part of the labyrinth that leads from the oval window is a bony, snail-shaped structure called the *cochlea*. The cochlea contains auditory liquids that the vibrations travel through. In the cochlea is a sensitive auditory receptor called the *organ of Corti*. Tiny hair cells in the organ of Corti receive vibrations from the auditory liquids and relay the sound waves to auditory nerve fibers, which end in the auditory center of the cerebral cortex. It is there that these impulses are interpreted and "heard."

Tympanic membrane comes from the Greek *tympanon*, meaning "drum," because it resembles a drum (hence *eardrum*). *Stapes*, Latin for "stirrup," was named, not surprisingly, for its stirrup-like shape.

Demystifying deafness

Deafness is diminished or total loss of hearing, and there are two types.

Conductive hearing loss is caused by obstruction of the path travelled by the sound waves from the external ear to the inner ear. Examples could be build-up of ear wax (cerumen), or a foreign body lodged in the external auditory meatus. Conductive deafness can be treated by removal of the obstruction.

Sensorineural deafness results from the damage to the auditory nerve or cochlea, preventing nerve stimuli from reaching the brain from the inner ear. This can occur with age but also can be caused by loud noises from machinery, music, tremors, infection, or injury. Hearing aids can help in treating sensorineural deafness. However, if a hearing aid is not successful, cochlear implants may be needed to have hearing restored.

The ear is also an organ of *equilibrium* or balance. The three organs within the inner ear responsible for equilibrium are the *semicircular canals*, the *saccule*, and *utricle*. These organs contain a fluid called *endolymph*, as well as sensitive hair cells. The fluid and hair cells fluctuate with movement of the head and transmit impulses in nerve fibers leading to the brain. Messages are then sent to muscles throughout the body so that equilibrium (balance) is maintained.

The Nose

Our sense of smell, though not as important to humans as it is to animals, basically performs the same purpose. An animal's sense of smell is acute, as it warns of danger and acts as a guide in finding food. We aren't so different, more in degree than in kind — we can smell smoke before we see fire, and we all know about smelling good food.

The *olfactory epithelium* of the nose is the organ of smell. Olfactory (*olfact* refers to smell) receptors in the *root* (area between eyes) of the nose are stimulated by odor, and chemical messages are transmitted to the *olfactory bulb* and sent to the olfactory centers of the brain. We can smell six basic odors: fruity, flowery, spicy, burned, putrid, and resin. The sense of smell acts to complement the taste sense, which is why a clogged nose with a head cold interferes with smelling, and food loses its flavors.

(Because this chapter is about the special senses, we're really dealing with the nose's sense of smell. The mucus, hairs, and septum (the part separating the nostrils) have nothing to do with smelling. But, if you're so inclined to know more about them, check out Chapter 17.)

You have 60 million olfactory epithelium cells in your nose. Way to go!

The Mouth

The organs of taste are the *taste buds*, found on the tongue and in the mucous membranes lining the soft palate of the mouth.

We can distinguish only four primary tastes: sweet, sour, salty, and bitter; the variety of tastes we experience are mixtures of the four, much as the colors we see are mixtures of the three primary colors. For food to initiate the sensation of taste, it must be dissolved by saliva, which is why taste buds are in a moist area. Much that we think we taste is really smelled, and the taste depends on the odor. Our sense of taste and smell work together in this way.

You have 10,000 taste bud *papillae* on surface of your tongue.

The Touch Receptor

The skin (which is the body's largest organ) is our only *touch receptor*. Touch sensation, often referred to as *light pressure*, varies in different parts of the body. The sensitive areas are those that provide the most information about ourselves and the external environment. Lips and fingers have the most receptors, in a concentrated area, which is why we use them more than, say, our elbows, to touch and identify objects.

The *dermis* of the skin has nerve endings that act as the receptors. They sense hot and cold, pain, pressure, and touch. The nervous system carries messages to the brain when changes to temperature, injury, or pressure occurs. For more information on your skin, see Chapter 14.

Sensory Root Words

Get ready. The sensory systems use a *lot* of root words, prefixes, and suffixes, and with good reason. Consider that this set of systems includes some delicate and sophisticated body parts: eyes, ears, nose, mouth, and skin. It's no wonder that we need a lot of combining forms and roots to fully describe the wonders of the senses.

We'll start small with taste, smell, and touch in Table 15-1. Then you can move on to the eyes and ears, which are slightly more complicated.

Table 15-1	Forms of Taste, Smell, and Touch
Word or Word Part	*What It Means*
A- or an-	Without, or lack of
Dys-	Difficult or uncomfortable
Geusia	Taste
Hyper-	Excess – more than normal
Hypo-	Less than normal
-itis	Inflammation
Osmia	Smell

See, that wasn't so hard! Now that you have your feet wet (or nose, as it may be), you can move on to the eye, which has about a gazillion (okay, maybe that's an exaggeration) root words and combining forms. Check it out in Table 15-2.

Table 15-2	Visual Roots
Root Word	*What It Means*
Aque/o	Water
Blephar/o	Eyelid
Conjunctiv/o	Conjunctiva (membrane lining eyelids)
Core/o, cor/o	Pupil
Corne/o	Cornea
Dacry/o	Tear, tear duct
Dipl/o	Double
Emmetr/o	In due measure
Glauc/o	Gray
Ir/o, irid/o	Iris (colored portion of the eye)
Is/o	Equal
Kerat/o	Cornea
Lacrim/o	Tear, tear duct
Mi/o	Smaller, less
Mydri/o	Wide

(continued)

Table 15-2 (continued)

Root Word	What It Means
Ocul/o	Eye
Ophthalm/o	Eye (ophthalmologist, specialist in eye disorders)
Opt/o	Eye, vision
Phac/o, phak/o	Crystalline lens
Phot/o	Light
Presby/o	Old age
Pupill/o	Pupil
Retin/o	Retina
Scler/o	Sclera (white of the eye)
Uve/o	Iris, ciliary body, and choroids
Vitre/o	Glassy
Xer/o	Dry

A prefix and a few suffixes associated with sight include the ones in Table 15-3.

Table 15-3 — Visual Prefix and Suffixes

Prefix or Suffix	What It Means
Bi- or bin-	Two
-chalasis	Relaxation
-ician	One who
-metrist	Specialist in the measurement of
-opia	Vision (condition)
-ory	Pertaining to
-oscopy	Visual examination of internal cavity using a scope
-plasty	Surgical repair or reconstruction
-tropia	To turn

The labyrinth of your ear is a complicated place with twists, turns, and many working parts. As such, medical professionals have a lot of words to use when describing what goes on in there. Thankfully, though, the list of root words and suffixes (no prefixes here) is fairly compact. Listen up to Tables 15-4 and 15-5.

Table 15-4	Listening to Your Roots
Root Word	*What It Means*
Acous/o, Acou/o	Hearing
Audi/o	Hearing
Aur/o, Aur/i	Ear
Bar/o	Pressure, weight
Cerumin/o	Cerumen (ear wax)
Mastoid/o	Mastoid process (process of temporal bone behind the ear)
Myring/o	Eardrum, tympanic membrane
Ot/o	Ear
Staped/o	Stapes (third ossicle of middle ear)
Tympan/o	Eardrum, middle ear

Strangely, as we mentioned, there really aren't any ear-related prefixes to discuss. There are, however, several suffixes to keep you busy in Table 15-5.

Table 16-5	Hearing Suffixes
Suffix	*What It Means*
-cusis	Hearing
-gram	Record
-itis	Inflammation
-metry	Process of measuring
-otomy	Process of cutting into
-phonia	Sound
-rrhea	Discharge or flow
-scope	Instrument used to visually examine

It's All Related: More Anatomical Terms

Holy lists and sidebars, Batman! As you can see, this chapter is chock-full of words you need to know about the senses. What can you say? There is a lot of ground to cover with these, but very important, parts of your body. Just the eye alone gets its own list of extra vocabulary words here (Table 15-6). Get your flashcards and markers ready to rock.

Table 15-6	Sight Words, Literally
Word	*What It Means*
Accommodation	Adjustment of the lens to focus on the retina
Astigmatism	Defective curvature of the refractive surface of the eye
Binocular	Pertaining to two or both eyes
Blepharitis	Inflammation of the eyelid
Corneal	Pertaining to the cornea
Conjunctivitis	Inflammation of the conjunctiva
Diplopia	Double vision
Hyperopia	Farsightedness
Keratitis	Inflammation of the cornea
Keratometer	Instrument used to measure the curvature of the cornea, used when fitting contact lenses
Myopia	Nearsightedness
Nyctalopia	Poor vision at night or in faint light
Ophthalmalgia	Pain in the eye
Ophthalmic	Pertaining to the eye
Ophthalmologist	Physician who specializes in ophthalmology
Ophthalmology	The study of diseases and treatment of the eye
Ophthalmoscope	Instrument used for visual examination of the interior of eye
Optician	One who is skilled in filling prescriptions for lenses
Optometer	Instrument used to measure power and range of vision
Optometrist	A health professional who prescribes corrective lenses
Optometry	Measurement of visual acuity and prescribing of corrective lenses
Presbyopia	Impaired vision as a result of aging

Hopefully your head isn't spinning from vocabulary overload at this point. If so, take a breather before continuing on to the next big list of words, which is a big ol' bunch of aural word salad (Table 15-7).

Table 15-7	An Earful of Vocabulary
Word	*What It Means*
Acoumeter	Instrument used to measure hearing
Audiologist	One who specializes in audiology
Audiology	The study of hearing
Aural	Pertaining to the ear
Otologist	A physician who studies and treats diseases of the ear
Otology	The study of the ear
Otorhinolaryngology (ENT)	The study and treatment of diseases and disorders of ear, nose, and throat
Otorhinolaryngologist	A physician specialized in otorhinolaryngology
Otorrhea	Discharge from the ear
Otoscope	Instrument used for visual examination of the ear
Purulent otitis media	Inflammation of the middle ear, resulting in the build-up of pus
Serous otitis media	Inflammation of inner ear, resulting in a build-up of watery fluid
Tympanometer	Instrument to measure middle ear function
Tympanometry	Measurement of the movement of the tympanic membrane

Common Sensory Conditions

Though it may seem obvious, it deserves being said. Most of the conditions associated with smell and taste involve the body's inability to perform those sensory tasks. Having trouble smelling your spring flowers? Can't taste your famous five-alarm chili? Chances are that it's dues to one of these conditions:

- **Ageusia:** Lack of or impairment of taste
- **Anosmia:** Absence of sense of smell
- **Dysgeusia:** Abnormal or perverted sense of taste
- **Dysosmia:** Impaired sense of smell
- **Hypergeusia:** Excessive or acute sense of taste
- **Osmesis:** The process of smelling

As usual, the eye is infinitely more complicated than, say, your tongue. So it stands to reason that there are many more possible conditions associated with your sense of sight. Though common, all of these conditions are serious and should not be taken lightly. They are

- **Chalazion:** Small, hard mass on the eyelid due to oil gland enlargement
- **Esotropia:** A type of strabismus (one eye turns inward, cross-eyed)
- **Exotropia:** A type of strabismus (one eye turns outward)
- **Glaucoma:** Increased intraocular pressure
- **Hemianopia (hemianopsia):** Loss of one half of the visual field (the space of vision of eye)
- **Hordeolum (sty or stye):** An infection of the oil gland of the eyelid
- **Nystagmus:** Involuntary, rapid movements of the eyeball
- **Retinal detachment:** The retina, or part of it, becomes separated from the choroid layer
- **Strabismus:** Abnormal deviation of the eye; also called a squint

Moving on to the other complicated sense organ, the ear, you can see that quite a few of these conditions result in some from of hearing loss. Some are unavoidable, but thankfully, some of these can be avoided by exercising good hygiene and staying away from rock concerts (or at least wearing ear plugs).

- **Macrotia:** Abnormal enlargement of the pinna (excessively large ears)
- **Microtia:** Abnormally small pinna (excessively small ears)
- **Myringitis:** Inflammation of tympanic membrane
- **Otalgia:** Pain in the ear (earache)
- **Otitis externa:** Inflammation of the outer ear; also known as swimmer's ear
- **Otitis media:** Infection of the middle ear

- **Tympanitis:** Inflammation of the middle ear (otitis media)

- **Serous otitis media:** Inflammation of the inner ear without infection

- **Suppurative otitis media:** Bacterial infection of middle ear

- **Tinnitus:** Ringing sound in ears; cause unknown, may be associated with chronic otitis, myringitis, or labyrinthitis

- **Vertigo:** Sensation of irregular or whirling motion, of body or external objects, due to severe disturbance of equilibrium organs in the labyrinth

Finding the Culprit: Sensory Diseases and Pathology

Once again, the eyes and ears rule. These two areas are just as susceptible to pathological diseases as any other site on the body. Some of the greatest hits include

- **Acoustic neuroma:** Benign tumor in acoustic nerve in the brain causing tinnitus, vertigo, and decreased hearing

- **Cataract:** Clouding of the lens, causing decreased vision

- **Cholesteatoma:** Collection of skin cells and cholesterol in a sac in the middle ear

- **Diabetic retinopathy:** Retinal effects of diabetic mellitus

- **Macular degeneration:** Deterioration of the *macula lutea* of the retina

- **Meniere's disease or syndrome:** Vertigo, hearing loss, nausea and tinnitus, leading to progressive deafness caused by rapid violent firing of the fibers of the auditory nerves

- **Otosclerosis:** Hardening of the bony tissue of the labyrinth causing hearing loss and progressive deafness

- **Presbycusis:** Hearing loss occurring with old age

- **Retinitis pigmentosa:** Progressive retinal sclerosis and atrophy; an inherited disease associated with decreased vision and night blindness (nyctalopia)

Testing, Testing: Sensory Radiology and Diagnostic tests

Your physician will want to run a battery of tests if you ever encounter problems with any of your senses, particularly with the eyes and ears. There is no doubt that your body and brain get a huge percentage of incoming information from these two sense organs alone, and if you lose the capability for either, your entire world will change. These are tests to take very seriously:

✔ **Audiogram:** The graphed test results of audiometry

✔ **Audiometry:** An audiometer delivers acoustic stimuli of specific frequencies to determine hearing for each frequency using an instrument to measure acuity of hearing

✔ **Diathermy:** The use of high-frequency electrical current to coagulate blood vessels within the eye

✔ **Gonioscopy:** Involves the examination of the angle of the anterior chamber of the eye to diagnose glaucoma

✔ **Laser photocoagulation:** Used to treat diabetic retinopathy and senile macular degeneration

✔ **Ophthalmoscopy:** Visual examination of the interior of the eye

✔ **Otoscopy:** Visual examination of the ear with an otoscope

✔ **Proetz test:** Test for acuity of smell

✔ **Slit lamp biomicroscopy:** A microscopic study of the cornea, conjunctiva, iris, lens, and vitreous humor

✔ **Tonometry:** Measurement of the tension or pressure within the eye

✔ **Tuning fork test (Weber's test):** A vibration source (tuning fork) is placed on forehead to note sound perception on right, left, or midline

✔ **Visual acuity:** Test of clarity or clearness of vision; reading the Snedden eye chart of black letters in decreasing size with the chart at a distance of 20 feet. 20/20 vision indicates that letters can be clearly seen at that distance. 20/50 vision indicates the eye is able to see at 20 feet what it is supposed to be able to see at 50 feet.

✔ **Visual field test:** Test measures the area within which objects can be seen when the eye is fixed and looking straight ahead

Paging Dr. Terminology: Surgeries and Procedures

Thankfully, there is something that can be done about a lot of those common eye conditions and diseases. Surgical procedures for the eye have improved dramatically over time and often involve less invasive procedures. Either way, though, you might want to call a cab afterwards.

- **Blepharoplasty:** Surgical repair of the eyelid
- **Cataract surgery:** To remove the lens when a cataract has formed
- **Cryoextraction of a cataract:** This method uses a cold probe to the anterior surface of the lens to lift the lens out as it adheres to the probe
- **Enucleation:** Surgical removal of the eye
- **Keratoplasty:** This procedure, also called a *corneal transplant*, involves replacement of a section of an opaque cornea with a normal transparent cornea in an effort to restore vision.
- **Phacoemulsification:** Removal of cataract
- **Phacoemulsification of a cataract:** Involves using ultrasonic vibration to break up portions of the lens. The lens is aspirated through the ultrasonic probe.
- **Scleroplasty:** Repair of the sclera
- **Vitrectomy:** Diseased vitreous humor is removed and replaced with clear solution.

Procedures for the ear are a bit more invasive, obviously, because so much is going on within the labyrinth of canals inside your head. Some of the most common clinical and surgical procedures for the ear include

- **Fenestration:** Forming an opening into labyrinth to restore hearing
- **Labyrinthectomy:** Excision of the labyrinth
- **Mastoidectomy:** Excision of the mastoid bone
- **Mastoidotomy:** Incision into the mastoid bone
- **Myringoplasty:** Surgical repair of the tympanic membrane
- **Myringotomy:** Incision of the tympanic membrane performed to release pus and relieve pressure in the middle ear

✔ **Stapedectomy:** Excision of the stapes

✔ **Tympanoplasty:** Surgical repair of the eardrum

✔ **Tympanectomy:** Surgical removal of the eardrum

Terminology RX: Sensory Pharmacology

Antibiotics, corticosteroids, and antivirals are often used to treat both ear and eye infections. Most eye infections are treated with *topical drugs* (ointments, liquids or creams, *topical* meaning applied directly to the area, eye drops, ear drops, and antibiotics). Most *ophthalmic antibiotics* are classified as topical applications, as are *corticosteroids* used to treat inflammation often after surgery, trauma, or chemical contact. Here are some other sensory meds to know:

✔ **Balanced salt solution** (BSS) is used during eye surgery to irrigate and wash the eye.

Do not confuse BSS with *normal saline*, as they are not the same. BSS is a registered ophthalmic preparation used in eye surgeries, a slightly different compound than normal saline, which is a sterile salt solution.

✔ **Beta blockers** are used to treat glaucoma.

✔ **Mydriatic drugs** (drugs that dilate the pupil) are used at eye examinations.

✔ **Silver nitrate** is commonly used as a topical anti-infective agent, administered to eyes of newborn infants to prevent infection.

Part IV
Let's Get Some Physiology Terminology

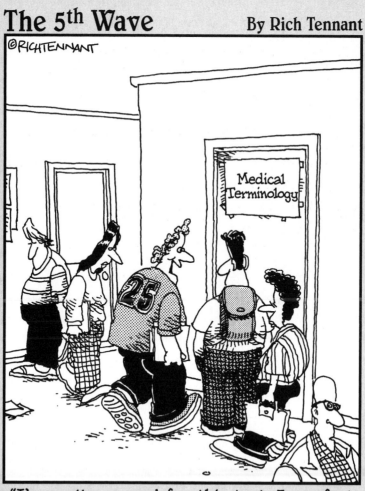

The 5th Wave   By Rich Tennant

Medical Terminology

"I'm really pumped for this test. I can feel the watcha ma call it flowing through those little round tube things in my body."

In this part . . .

This section goes even deeper into body systems and how they operate. Chapter 16 keeps the beat moving with a discussion about your cardiovascular system. Chapter 17 introduces you to the respiratory system. Chapter 18 covers the voyage your food takes through the gastrointestinal system, whereas Chapter 19 shows you words associated with cleaning out your body via the endocrine system. And Chapter 20 shows you medical terms that deal with your nervous system.

Chapter 16

The Heart of the Matter: The Cardiovascular and Lymphatic Systems

In This Chapter

▶ Discovering how your heart, blood vessels, and lymph nodes work together

▶ Memorizing root words, prefixes, and suffixes appropriate to these systems

▶ Discussing common cardiovascular and lymphatic conditions and diseases

▶ Getting to the heart of the correct terms to use when diagnosing problems

▶ Understanding how to communicate terms used in surgeries and procedures

*E*ver wonder how we have fresh, clean water to drink? A vast network of lakes, reservoirs, pumping and purification stations, and pipes ultimately bring us the life force that is water. We, in turn, use it for drinking, cooking, cleaning, and a multitude of tasks.

Your cardiovascular system is not so different. Consider your heart as the big central pumping station that supplies the rest of your body with valuable liquid — mainly, blood. Blood carries oxygen and nutrients to body tissues and collects carbon dioxide and waste materials to be eliminated. You can think of the complementary lymphatic system as the wastewater treatment facility that cleans and purifies what was once useless into clear, clean fluid.

How the Cardiovascular System Works

Let's try another metaphor. Although the heart is the main character in this sweeping drama called *Your Body*, it couldn't do its work without a strong cast of supporting characters: blood, blood cells, and vessels. The separate but complementary lymphatic system works like ushers at a play, guiding no-longer-useful folks out at the end of the show. None of these components can work alone. They are a merry band of players who must share the spotlight.

The main organ of the circulatory (another name for cardiovascular) system is the *heart*, of course, and its main job is making the blood flow freely through your veins. By pumping, the heart creates pressure that forces the blood to move throughout the body via a channel system of *arteries* and *veins*. That system reaches from the center of your chest out to the nether regions of your appendages and back again, insuring that life-giving and sustaining blood cells are carried through your entire body.

The lymphatic system works to complement the actions of the cardiovascular system by carrying *lymph fluid* through the body via a system similar to veins. The lymph fluid flows forward through a grouping of *vessels*, *ducts*, and *nodes* that filter the fluid before it re-enters the bloodstream. In this chapter, you find out more about the individual components of these two powerful systems and get to know the specific terminology associated with both.

An adult human's normal heart rate is 70–80 beats per minute. A child's is 100–120, an elephant's about 25, a mouse's 700, and a canary's heart beats about 1,000 times per minute. Your heart beats around 100,000 times a day, pumping $2^{1}/_{2}$ ounces with each contraction. That's 5 quarts a minute, 75 gallons per hour, 1,800 gallons a day, and 657,000 gallons per year.

Greek plays a role in the roots of the word for heart, *cardium*. This word, which you'll get to know quite well in this chapter, is taken from the Greek word *kardia*. *Cardium* takes on other identities in the commonly known forms of *cardi* and *cardio*. But make no mistake, it's all the same root.

Now, meet the individual players responsible for the pumping of the red stuff that keeps you going every day. Each has its own special function and terminology to go along with it. If watching ER is your only entrée into the world of medical terminology, fear not and consider this section your crash course in all things cardiovascular.

The heart

To take a tour of the heart, consider three components: layers, chambers, and valves. Together, these elements form the most powerful muscle in the body. Located to the left of the midline of your chest's center, this muscle, about the size of your fist, pumps a continuous stream of life-giving blood through your blood vessels.

Figure 16-1 illustrates the heart.

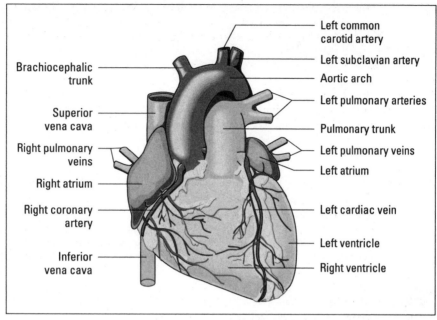

Brachiocephalic trunk

Superior vena cava

Right pulmonary veins

Right atrium

Right coronary artery

Inferior vena cava

Left common carotid artery

Left subclavian artery

Aortic arch

Left pulmonary arteries

Pulmonary trunk

Left pulmonary veins

Left atrium

Left cardiac vein

Left ventricle

Right ventricle

Figure 16-1:
Anterior view of the heart.

From LifeARTS®, Super Anatomy 1, ©2002, Lippincott Williams & Wilkins

The heart is enclosed in a fluid-filled sac called the *pericardium*, located in the chest cavity just to the left of the midline. It consists of three major layers, each one performing a unique job in the day-to-day activities of your most vital organ.

- ✔ **Endocardium:** *Endo-* is the Greek prefix for "within." This is the inner layer of the heart, lining the chambers and covering the valves.

- ✔ **Epicardium:** *Epi-* is the Greek prefix for "on." This is the outer layer of the heart.

- ✔ **Myocardium:** *Myo-* is the Greek prefix meaning "muscle." This is the actual heart muscle and makes up the thick middle layer.

The four hollow places in the heart are called *chambers*. There are two types of chamber:

- ✔ **Atrium:** *Atrium* is taken from the Greek word *atrion*, meaning "hall." The right and left *atria* (*atrium* is the singular form) are the two upper heart chambers serving as receiving stations for blood. Valves connect each atrium to the ventricles below.

- ✔ **Ventricles:** *Ventricle* is taken from the Latin word *venter*, meaning "little belly." The right and left ventricles are thick, lower chambers and are responsible for pumping blood. The atria receive blood from the body, and the ventricles pump blood back out into the body.

The four heart chambers are separated by membranes called *septa* (plural of *septum*).

- ✔ **Interatrial septum** separates the two atria.
- ✔ **Interventricular septum** separates the two ventricle chambers.

Valves are the gatekeepers of the heart, making sure the blood flows in the correct direction. They let a specific amount of blood into each chamber and don't allow it to flow backwards. The beauty of valve terminology is that the name of each valve gives you a clue to its make-up.

- ✔ **Bicuspid valve (also called mitral):** The *bi-* prefix shows you that this valve has two flaps.
- ✔ **Pulmonary semilunar valve and aortic semilunar valve:** Both have a half-moon shape, thus being named from *semi* (part) and *lunar* (moon).
- ✔ **Tricuspid valve:** *Tri-* indicates this valve has three flaps, keeping blood moving forward.

Blood vessels

The vast network of blood vessels (made up of arteries and arterioles, veins and venules, and capillaries) begins at the heart and spans out through the entire body to the far reaches of the fingertips and toes. Together, these different types of vessels work to carry blood pumped by the heart through the body.

Arteries take care of clean, oxygenated blood. *Veins* handle the movement of deoxygenated blood. Your little friends, the *capillaries*, serve as mini bridges between the two types of vessels.

Arterial system

The *arterial system* is composed of arteries and *arterioles* (smaller arteries). The Greek *aer* is the basis for the word *artery*, meaning "air." Combined with *terein*, meaning "to keep," you get the word *artery*. Starting with the largest artery, the *aorta*, the arteries carry oxygenated blood away from the heart to the arterioles, and then on to the capillaries, where the exchange of gases (oxygen and carbon dioxide) takes place.

The *pulmonary artery*, with its two branches, is the exception of the arterial world. Instead of carrying oxygen-filled blood to other parts of the body, its branches carry oxygen-deprived blood to the right and left lungs.

Venous system

The venous system is made up of veins and *venules* (little veins). The veins are the workhorses of the vessel system, carrying oxygen-depleted blood back to the heart. The journey ends with the blood from the head and upper body being returned to the heart via the body's largest veins, the *superior vena cava,* and from the lower body via the *inferior vena cava,* received into the right atrium. The pulmonary veins carry oxygen-rich blood from the lungs back to the heart.

Capillaries

If you look at a map of the blood vessel system, you see that capillaries are incredibly small and look tiny, like hair. It's no accident, then, that the word *capillary* is Latin for "hair-like." These super-tiny vessels (one cell thick, to be exact) bridge the gap between arterioles and venules to keep blood flowing in a continuous motion.

Figure 16-2 illustrates capillary exchange.

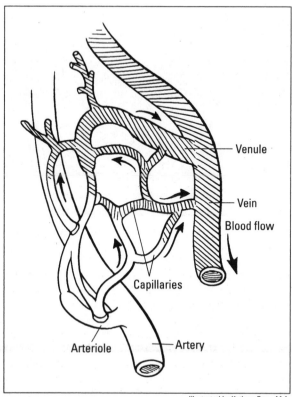

Figure 16-2:
Artery, vein, and capillary exchange.

Illustrated by Kathryn Born, M.A.

Following the trail of blood

A great way to remember much of the terminology associated with the heart is to think more about the path the blood takes each time it makes a trip through the vast muscle.

The *rule of two* will get you started. Remember that the heart has two different types of chambers: ventricles and atria, which both contract at the same time. Similarly, the blood travels through two paths: the arterial system for sending oxygen-rich blood out and the venous system for bringing oxygen-poor blood back.

Next, try to think of the blood's path as "The Hokey Pokey." Remember? "You put your right

foot in. You put your right foot out," and so on. Think of where the blood goes in and out, and you can click through around fifteen cardiovascular terms. Let's follow it:

Left ventricle > aorta > arteries > arterioles > capillaries of body tissues > back through venules > veins > superior/inferior venae cavae > right atrium > right ventricle > pulmonary artery > alveoli of the lungs > lung capillaries > pulmonary veins > left atrium > left ventricle . . . and it begins again. Feel free to put this path to the music of your choice and sing along!

Blood

There's more to the make-up of your blood than the obvious red blood cells. A large percentage of your blood is actually made up of *plasma*, which is, in turn, largely composed of water. The red and white cells, plus *platelets*, make up the rest of your ever-flowing life force. Here's a bit more about what makes up your blood:

- ✔ **Plasma:** Mostly water, a small percentage of plasma is composed of proteins, nutrients, waste, and gas. *Albumin, fibrinogen,* and *immunoglobin* are all proteins found in plasma.

- ✔ **Platelets:** The body's little firemen. Platelets are always putting out "fires" in the body by beginning the clotting process and putting a stop to any blood escaping from a compromised vessel.

- ✔ **Red blood cells:** Also known as *erythrocytes*, these cells contain *hemoglobin*, a protein composed of molecules containing *globin* and *iron*. Red blood cells carry oxygenated blood throughout the body.

- ✔ **White blood cells:** Called *leukocytes*, these are the double agents of the cardiovascular system. They work as the body's homemade antibiotics, fighting germs in both the bloodstream and in tissue fluid and lymph fluid.

Path of the blood

Veins carry blood back to the heart via the superior and inferior venae cavae. The *superior* (meaning "near the top") *vena cava* takes blood from the upper body to the right atrium; the *inferior* (meaning situated below) *vena cava* carries blood from the lower body to the right atrium, which then empties the blood into the right ventricle. The ventricle contracts, expelling the blood into the pulmonary artery.

Pulmon is the Latin word for "lung."

The pulmonary arteries carry the blood through to the lungs where it is *oxygenated*. From there, the pulmonary veins carry the oxygenated blood back to the left atrium, which then moves the blood into the left ventricle, which pumps the blood into the aorta.

Thank good old Aristotle for the word *aorta*, meaning "that which is hung." The philosopher named it so because of the upside-down, hanging curve of the artery.

Cardiac cycle

All this pumping and moving of blood comes down to rhythm. The *cardiac cycle* is controlled by the heart's natural pacemaker, the *sinoatrial (SA) node*. The rhythmic pulsations conduct through the *AV node*, down the *AV bundle* (also known as the *bundle of His*), through the *Purkinje fibers*, jump-starting contraction of the ventricles.

There are two phases in the cardiac cycle:

- ✔ **Diastole** is the resting period, when the heart rests and fills with blood.
- ✔ **Systole** is the period when ventricles contract and send blood out, causing pressure on the walls of the arteries during the heart's contraction.

Both words share a Greek root, *stole*, meaning "to send." The difference lies in the prefix. *Dia-* means "apart," whereas *sy-* means "together."

How the Lymphatic System Works

Most directly associated with immunity, we discuss the lymphatic system in the same chapter as the cardiovascular system due to the similar make-up of the system and the fact that, once cleaned by the lymph nodes, lymphatic fluid is released directly into the bloodstream. Lymph vessels are arranged in a similar pattern as the blood vessels, but work to clear the body of impurities.

Lymphatic vessels

Lymphatic vessels borrow their name from the fluid they pump, called, not surprisingly, *lymph fluid*. Curiously, at the heart of the word *lymph* is the Greek *nymph*, a term used to describe a beautiful maiden. The word eventually took on Latin roots, when the *n* was replaced with *l*. Because lymph fluid is a clear, clean fluid, and *lymph* rhymes with *nymph*, the transition was apparent to Latin wordsmiths.

The lymphatic vessels interlace with blood vessels to carry clean lymphatic fluid through the body. They collect the proteins and water, which continually filter out of the blood into tissue fluid, and return to the blood. The proteins and water filter out of the blood and escape into tissue fluid. The lymphatic vessels pick up the proteins and water from the tissues and return them to the blood.

Lymph nodes, also called "glands"

Shaped much like small beans, the *lymph nodes* are located throughout the body. We discuss what the nodes do later in the chapter, but here is the low-down on the location of these helpful little guys. Lymph nodes are located in several regions of the body. Depending on where they are, lymph nodes are known by different names, including

- **Axillary:** Underarm and upper chest
- **Cervical:** Neck
- **Inguinal:** Groin

Figure 16-3 illustrates a lymph node.

Lymphatic System

The lymphatic system is largely responsible for creating an immunity barrier by developing and distributing *lymphocytes,* a type of WBC (white blood cell) throughout the body. Lymphocytes are our little buddies, which you read about earlier. The lymph nodes release these *lymphocytes* and remove or destroy *antigens* (foreign substances that invoke an immune response) that circulate through the blood and lymphatic vessels.

Lymph fluid enters the node, filters through *sinuses* within the node, and drains through a single exit vessel. Consider it a one-way ticket for lymph fluid to get into the bloodstream. This filter system cleans out all of the yucky stuff: bacteria, foreign particles, and those naughty malignant cells. The lymph nodes also destroy invading cells and particles in a process known as *phagocytosis*. The *thoracic duct* (there is only one) is the largest vessel of the lymph system. It collects lymph from the body below the diaphragm and from left side of body above the diaphragm.

The spleen, tonsils, and thymus are accessory organs of this system. The *spleen* enlarges with infectious diseases and decreases in size in old age. Some phagocytosis takes place in the spleen. The *tonsils* filter out bacteria and foreign matter. The *thymus* produces cells that destroy foreign substances.

Figure 16-4 illustrates the lymphatic system.

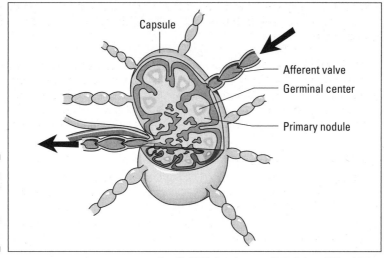

Capsule

Afferent valve

Germinal center

Primary nodule

Figure 16-3:
Anatomy
of a lymph
node, cross
section.

From LifeARTS®, Super Anatomy 1, ©2002, Lippincott Williams & Wilkins

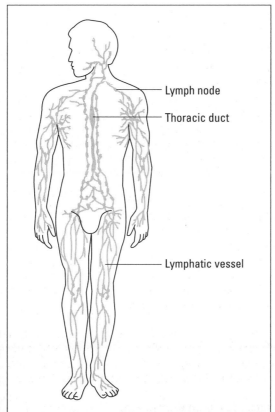

Lymph node

Thoracic duct

Lymphatic vessel

Figure 16-4:
The
lymphatic
system.

From LifeARTS®, Super Anatomy 1, ©2002, Lippincott Williams & Wilkins

Cardiovascular and Lymphatic Root Words

Now that you've gotten to know the specific parts of the cardiovascular and lymphatic systems a bit better, it's time to put your expertise into practice. Table 16-1 lists cardio roots, prefixes, and suffixes. It also gives an example medical term for each.

Table 16-1	Breaking Down Your Cardio Words	
Root Word	**What It Means**	**Example**
Aort/o	Aorta	Aortic
Angi/o	Vessel	Angiogram
Arteri/o	Artery	Arteriosclerosis
Arteriol/o	Arteriole	Arteriolitis
Atri/o, atri/a	Atrium	Atrioventricular
Ather/o	Yellow plaque or fatty substance	Atherosclerosis
Cardi/o	Heart	Cardiomegaly
Coron/o	Heart	Coronary
Ox/o, ox/i	Oxygen	Oximeter
Phleb/o	Vein	Phlebitis
Pulmon/o	Lung	Pulmonary
Scler/o	Hardening	Sclerotherapy
Thromb/o	Clot	Thrombus
Valv/o, valvul/o	Valve	Valvular
Vas/o	Vessel	Vasoconstriction
Ven/o	Vein	Venotomy
Venul/o	Venule	Venulitis
Ventricul/o	Ventricle	Ventricular
Prefix or Suffix	**What It Means**	**Example**
Brady	Slow	Bradycardia
Tachy	Fast	Tachycardia
-graph	Instrument used to record	Electrocardiograph
-graphy	Process of recording	Electrocardiography
-gram	Picture or finished record	Electrocardiogram

Table 16-2 lists lymphatic roots and suffixes.

Table 16-2	Breaking Down Your Lymphatic Roots
Root Word	*What It Means*
Bas/o	Base (opposite of acid)
Eosin/o	Red, rosy
Erythr/o	Red
Granul/o	Granules
Hem/o, Hemat/o	Blood
Immun/o	Safe, protection
Kary/o	Nucleus
Leuk/o	White
Lymph/o	Lymph
Lymphaden/o	Lymph gland
Lymphangi/o	Lymph vessels
Neutr/o	Neither, neutral
Myel/o	Bone marrow
Mon/o	One, single
Morph/o	Shape, form
Nucle/o	Nucleus
Phleb/o	Vein
Spher/o	Globe or round
Sider/o	Iron
Splen/o	Spleen
Thromb/o	Clot
Thym/o	Thymus
Suffix	*What It Means*
-apheresis	Removal
-blast	Immature
-cytosis	Condition of cells
-emia	Blood condition
-globin	Protein
-globulin	Protein
-phoresis	Carrying, transmission
-poiesis	Formation
-stasis	Stop or control

Hundreds of medical terms can be created by using the roots, prefixes, and suffixes mentioned in the previous tables. In the next table, Table 16-3, we list some common cardiovascular and lymphatic vocabulary words.

Table 16-3	Cardiovascular and Lymphatic Vocabulary Words
Word	*What It Means*
Anticoagulant	Agent or drug that slows the clotting process
Aorta	Largest artery in the body
Atrium, Atria	Upper chambers of the heart
Auscultation	Hearing sounds in the body through a stethoscope
Blood pressure	Pressure exerted by blood against the vessel walls
Capillary	Smallest blood vessel
Cardiac	Pertaining to the heart
Cardiologist	Physician who studies and treats diseases of the heart
Cardiology	Study of the heart and its diseases
Cardiopulmonary resuscitation	(CPR) Emergency procedure consisting of artificial ventilation and external cardiac massage
Coronary arteries	The blood vessels that branch from the aorta to carry oxygen-rich blood to the heart muscle
Diastole	The relaxation phase of the heart beat
Endocardium	Inner lining of the heart
Erythrocyte	Red blood cell
Hematologist	Physician who studies and treats diseases of the blood
Hematology	Study of the blood
Hemolysis	Breakdown of blood
Hemostasis	Stoppage of bleeding
Immunoglobulins	Antibodies secreted by plasma cells
Leukocyte	White blood cell
Manometer	Instrument used to measure pressure of fluid

Word	What It Means
Mitral valve	Valve between the left atrium and left ventricle
Myelogenous	Produced by the bone marrow
Occlude	To be closed tightly
Percussion	Tapping of the body surface with fingers to determine density of the part beneath
Peyer's patches	Lymphatic filters located in the small intestine
Pulmonary arteries	Arteries carrying oxygen-poor blood from the heart to lungs
Pulmonary circulation	Flow of blood from the heart to the lungs and back to the heart
Pulmonary veins	Veins carrying oxygenated blood from the lungs to the heart
Sinoatrial (S-A) node	Pacemaker of the heart
Sphygmomanometer	Instrument used to measure blood pressure
Systemic circulation	Flow of blood from body cells to the heart and then back out of the heart to the cells
Systole	Contracting phase of the heartbeat
Thrombocyte	Clotting cell or platelet
Venae cavae	The largest veins in the body; the superior and inferior bring blood into the right atrium

Common Cardiovascular and Lymphatic Conditions

Some cardiovascular conditions pertain specifically to the heart and surrounding system of veins and arteries. First, let's consider what can ail some of the individual parts of the heart. *Aortic stenosis* is the narrowing of the aorta. *Endocarditis* is the inflammation of the inner lining of the heart, whereas *pericarditis* is an inflammation of the pericardial sac (pericardium).

Then there are conditions that involve the entire heart muscle, including *cardiomegaly*, enlargement of the heart, and *cardiomyopathy*, disease of the heart muscle. *Myocarditis* is an inflammation of the muscle of the heart. The two big daddies are — no surprise here — a *myocardial infarction*, also known as a heart attack, and good old *cardiac arrest*, the sudden cessation or stoppage of cardiac output and effective circulation. Don't forget *congestive heart failure*, *angina*, and *atrial fibrillation*.

Our blood travels through the superhighway of our arterial and venous systems, and it carries a lot of passengers, from oxygen to lymph. Because it is so multifaceted, the blood and its cells can harbor all sorts of conditions. Here is a sampling:

- ✔ **Anemia:** Lack of red blood cells

- ✔ **Dyscrasia:** Abnormal or pathological condition of the blood

- ✔ **Embolus (plural: emboli):** Also called an *embolism*, the sudden blockage of an artery by foreign material in the bloodstream, most often a blood clot but could be fat, an air bubble, or a clot of bacteria

- ✔ **Hemorrhage:** Rapid flow of blood

- ✔ **Hyperbilirubinemia:** Excessive amounts of bilirubin (a bile pigment excreted by the liver) in the blood

- ✔ **Hypercholesterolemia:** Excessive amounts of cholesterol (steroid alcohol that maintains membrane fluidity) in the blood

- ✔ **Hyperlipidemia:** Excessive amounts of fat in the blood

- ✔ **Hyperchromia:** Excessive pigmented red blood cells

- ✔ **Hypertension:** Blood pressure that is above normal range of 120/70

- ✔ **Hypotension:** Blood pressure that is below normal

- ✔ **Intermittent claudication:** Pain or discomfort in a body part caused by any activity which exerts the affected body part; often occurs in the calves while walking; a result of occlusive artery disease

- ✔ **Leukocytosis:** Marked increased in the number of white blood cells

- ✔ **Thrombolysis:** Breakdown of a clot that has formed in the blood

The lymphatic system has its own fair share of health issues. *Lymphadenitis* is an inflammation of lymph nodes. *Lymphedema* is an accumulation of fluid due to obstruction of lymphatic structures. And *splenomegaly* is an enlargement of the spleen.

Finding the Culprit: Cardiovascular and Lymphatic Diseases and Pathology

Pathology is a scary word, and for good reason. *Pathology* is the study of disease as it affects body tissue and function. Some conditions of the heart and lymph system are more serious and more risky than others. Although all conditions and diseases should be considered serious, these heavy hitters are ones that often require more in-depth procedures and treatments.

Why not start at — literally — the heart of the matter. Some pathological conditions affecting the heart and blood vessels include

- **Aneurysm**, a local widening of an artery, may be due to weakness in the arterial wall or breakdown of the wall due to atherosclerosis.

- **Angina pectoris** is an episode of chest pain due to temporary difference between the supply and demand of oxygen to the heart muscle.

- **Arterial hypertension** refers to high blood pressure. There are two types of hypertension: essential and secondary. In *essential hypertension*, the cause of the increased pressure is unknown or idiopathic. In *secondary hypertension*, there is an associated lesion, such as *nephritis*, *pyelonephritis* or *adenoma of the adrenal cortex,* which is responsible for the elevated blood pressure.

- **Bacterial endocarditis** is inflammation of the inner lining of the heart caused by bacteria.

  Keep the three types of cardiac arrhythmia straight. The *heart block* is a failure of proper conduction of impulses through the A-V node and can be overcome by implantation of an electric pacemaker. A *flutter* is rapid but regular contractions of the atria or ventricles, while *fibrillation* is rapid, random irregular contractions of the heart as high as 350+ beats per minute.

  Damage to the heart valves can produce lesions called vegetations, which may break off in the bloodstream as emboli or floating clots. Vegetation is an overgrowth of bacteria that gains a foothold on an injured valve, becoming fruitful and multiplying.

- **Cardiac arrhythmia** is an abnormal heart rhythm. Some examples include heart block, flutter, and fibrillation.

- **Congenital heart disease** refers to abnormalities in the heart at birth, resulting from some failure in the development of the fetus. *Coarctation of the aorta* is a narrowing of the aorta. Surgical treatment consists of removal of the constricted area with *end-to-end anastomosis* or joining together of the aortic segments.

- ✓ **Congestive heart failure** is a condition where the heart is unable to pump its required amount of blood . Blood accumulates in the lungs and liver. In severe cases, fluid can collect in the abdomen and legs or in the pulmonary air sacs (known as *pulmonary edema*). Congestive heart failure often develops gradually over the years and can be treated with drugs to strengthen the heart and diuretics to promote loss of fluid.

- ✓ **Coronary artery disease (CAD)** is a disease of arteries supplying blood to the heart. This is usually the result of *atherosclerosis*, the deposition of fatty compounds on the inner lining of the coronary arteries.

- ✓ **Heart murmur** refers to an extra heart sound heard between normal heart sounds. Murmurs are heard with the aid of a stethoscope and are caused by a valvular defect or disease, which disrupts the smooth flow of blood in the heart.

- ✓ **Hypertensive heart disease** is high blood pressure affecting the heart.

- ✓ **Mitral valve prolapse** is improper closure of the mitral valve when the heart is pumping blood.

- ✓ **Raynaud's phenomenon** is short episodes of discoloration and numbness in fingers and toes due to temporary constriction of arterioles. These may be triggered by cold temperature, stress, or smoking.

- ✓ **Rheumatic heart disease** is heart disease caused by rheumatic fever.

- ✓ **Varicose veins** are abnormally swollen veins usually occurring in the legs, due to damaged valves that fail to prevent the backflow of blood. The blood then collects in the veins, causing *distention*.

The blood itself can suffer from specific diseases and pathological conditions. Consider the diseases specific to both the red and white blood cells. *Anemia*, a common symptom, is a deficiency in erythrocytes or hemoglobin, can take several forms, including the following:

- ✓ **Aplastic anemia:** Failure of blood cell production due to absence of development and formation of bone marrow cells

- ✓ **Hemolytic anemia:** Reduction in red cells due to excessive destruction

- ✓ **Pernicious anemia:** Lack of mature erythrocytes due to inability to absorb vitamin B12

- ✓ **Sickle-cell anemia:** Hereditary condition in which distorted cells clump and block blood vessels

Other issues affecting the blood include *thalassemia*, an inherited defect in the ability to produce hemoglobin; *polycythemia vera*, a malignant condition associated with increased red blood cells: and *hemochromatosis*, excessive deposits of iron through the body. *Thalassemia* is usually found in patients of Mediterranean background.

The white blood cells often make people think of the "Big C," also known as cancer. This is for good reason, as the white cells have a lot to do with a very serious disease called *leukemia*. Leukemia, of course, is the kingpin of white blood cell pathology. It is, in simple terms, an excessive increase in white blood cells — a cancerous disease of the bone marrow with malignant leukocytes filling the marrow and bloodstream. Four forms of leukemia include:

- **Acute lymphocytic leukemia (ALL):** Seen most often in children and adolescents

- **Acute myelogenous leukemia (AML):** Derived from or originating in bone marrow

- **Chronic lymphocytic leukemia (CLL):** Occurs late in life and follows a slow, progressive course

- **Chronic myelogenous leukemia (CML):** Slowly progressive

All types of leukemia are treated with chemotherapy, using drugs that prevent cell division and selectively injure rapidly dividing cells. Effective treatment can lead to *remission*, or disappearance of signs of the disease. *Relapse* occurs when leukemia cells reappear in the blood and bone marrow, necessitating further treatment. Watch out for leukemia's nasty cousin, *multiple myeloma*. This is a malignant tumor of bone marrow in which malignant cells invade bone marrow and destroy bony structures.

Keep these two blood-clotting health issues in mind

- **Hemophilia** is excessive bleeding caused by a congenital lack of coagulation factor necessary for blood clotting.

- **Purpura** is a symptom caused by low platelets involving multiple pinpoint hemorrhages and accumulation of blood under the skin.

We couldn't leave our good friends in the lymphatic system out of the pathology discussion. Who knew that such small things like lymph nodes could be so prone to disease?

The lymph nodes themselves are the sites of many a showdown between good health and an extended hospital stay. *Hodgkin's disease* is a malignant tumor arising in lymphatic tissue such as lymph nodes and spleen. *Lymphosarcoma (lymphoma)* is a malignant tumor of lymph nodes that resembles Hodgkin's disease. Often referred to as *non-Hodgkin's lymphoma*, it affects lymph nodes, spleen, bone marrow, and other organs. *Burkitt's lymphoma* is a malignant tumor of lymph nodes usually affecting children and most common in central Africa.

HIV and AIDS

Perhaps the most serious diseases affecting the cardiovascular and lymphatic systems are HIV and AIDS.

HIV is also known as *human immunodeficiency virus*, the agent attacking the immune system and causing AIDS.

AIDS (*acquired immunodeficiency syndrome*) is a disease marked by a decrease in immune response in which the patient has severe depletion of *helper T-cell lymphocytes*. This could cause the patient to acquire unusual life-threatening infections and may develop tumors such as *Kaposi's sarcoma*, a skin and lymphoid cancer, or *lymphoma*.

Inflammation is another common trait of lymphatic system pathology. Sometimes those pesky lymph nodes just get too big for their britches in diseases like the following:

- **Lymphadenitis:** Inflammation of lymph nodes usually due to infection
- **Mononucleosis:** Acute infectious disease with enlarged lymph nodes and spleen due to increased numbers of lymphocytes and monocytes
- **Sarcoidosis:** Inflammatory disease in which small nodules form in lymph nodes and other organs

Testing, Testing: Cardiovascular and Lymphatic Radiology and Diagnostic Tests

Confirming the diagnosis of a condition or disease is a full-time job. Think about the insurance claim notices you receive every time you get blood work or a urine sample done. There is a lab test to diagnose practically anything that might ail you.

Lab tests for issues affecting the heart include *serum enzyme test or studies*, more commonly known as *cardiac enzymes*. During a myocardial infarction (heart attack), enzymes are released into the bloodstream from the dying heart muscle. These enzymes can be measured and are useful as evidence of an infarction. *Lipid tests* measure the amount of these substances in a blood sample. High levels of triglycerides and cholesterol can be associated with a greater risk of coronary atherosclerosis.

The *blood test* is the most common of all diagnostic tests. Blood work can help present a plethora of problems that not only affect blood but also major systems and organs. Another gold standard test is the *cardiac catheterization*, which involves inserting a long, thin tube, or catheter, into a blood vessel in the arm, neck, or groin that is then threaded to the heart to perform diagnostic testing such as pressure and patterns of blood flow.

Lipoprotein electrophoresis is a process in which *lipoproteins* (fat and protein molecules bound together) are physically separated from a blood sample. High levels of *low-density lipoprotein* (LDL) are associated with cholesterol and triglyceride deposits in arteries. High levels of *high-density lipoprotein* (HDL), containing less lipids, are found in someone with less evidence of atherosclerosis.

Remember *HDL* is the "happy" cholesterol in the blood. So, just remember *H* for "happy." *LDL* is the "bad" cholesterol. Remember *L* for "lousy."

Other laboratory blood tests include the following:

- **Antiglobulin test (Coombs' test)** determines whether erythrocytes are coated with antibody and useful in determining the presence of antibodies in infants of Rh-negative mothers. (Rh-negative is a blood type in which all Rh factors are lacking.)

- **Bleeding time** is measurement of the time it takes for a small puncture wound to stop bleeding; normal time is 8 minutes or less.

- **Coagulation time** is the time required for blood to clot in a test tube; normal time is less than 15 minutes.

- **ESR (erythrocyte sedimentation rate)** measures the speed at which erythrocytes settle out of plasma. The rate is altered in disease conditions such as infection, joint inflammation, and tumor.

- **Hemoglobin test** is the measurement of the amount of hemoglobin in a blood sample.

- **Platelet count** is the number of platelets per cubic millimeter of blood. Platelets normally average between 200,000–500,000 per cubic millimeter.

A common diagnostic test counts the red blood cells and/or the white blood cells. To remember the normal range for each, remember *RBC* (*really big count*) for RBC (red blood cells). The normal number is about 5 million per cubic millimeter. The *WBC* (*white blood cell count*) is much smaller, averaging between 5,000–10,000 per cubic millimeter.

- **Prothrombin time (PT)** is the ability of the blood to clot, used to follow patients taking blood thinners or anticoagulant drugs such as Coumadin.

- **White blood cell differential count** determines the number of different types of leukocytes, mature and immature, that are present in a blood sample.

Abbreviations: Keep it short and simple

You probably won't believe us, but saying all these terms over and over again can get tedious. Thankfully for those of you who must utter blood-related phrases on a daily basis, there are some handy-dandy abbreviations.

- ✔ **BP:** Blood pressure
- ✔ **CBC:** Complete blood count
- ✔ **DVT:** Deep vein thrombosis
- ✔ **Hct:** Hematocrit
- ✔ **Hgb or Hb:** Hemoglobin
- ✔ **PT:** Prothombin time
- ✔ **RBC:** Red blood cell count (erythrocytes)
- ✔ **WBC:** White blood cell count (leukocytes)

Paging Dr. Terminology: Cardiovascular and Lymphatic Surgeries and Procedures

So, what do you do about all of these conditions and diseases? Thankfully, there are almost as many possible surgeries and procedures as there are conditions and diseases. The clinical procedures for the cardiovascular system are many, so hunker down. The great majority of these directly involve the old ticker.

Electrocardiography is a record of the electricity flowing through the heart. Speaking of electricity, *cardioversion* or *defibrillation* is a treatment procedure whereby short discharges of electricity are applied across the chest to stop cardiac arrhythmia.

Angiocardiography is a procedure involving injection of contrast dye into the bloodstream followed by chest x-ray to determine the dimensions of the heart and large vessels. This is often used to diagnose an enlarged heart. Similarly, *digital subtraction angiography* can be used to get a closer look at the vessels. Video equipment and computer are used to produce x-rays of the blood vessels.

Other procedures focus on finding out more about how efficiently the heart is working. In *cardiac catheterization*, a catheter is introduced into a vein or artery and guided into the heart for purposes of detecting pressure and patterns of blood flow. The *cardiac scan* is when a radioactive substance is injected intravenously and its accumulation in the heart muscle is measured with a scanner.

The presence of areas of *ischemia* (deficiency of blood in a body part due to constriction or complete obstruction of a blood vessel) and myocardial infarction can be demonstrated on this scan. Everyone's favorite, the *stress test*, determines the body's response to physical exertion or stress. An *echocardiogram* and other measurements of blood pressure and breathing rate are taken while the patient is exercising usually jogging on a treadmill.

Other fun and exciting procedures include the following

- **Doppler flow study** uses ultrasound waves to determine the velocity of flow of blood within vessels.

- **Laser angioplasty** uses light amplification to stimulate emission of radiation or a laser beam to blocked arteries, especially in the legs.

- **Percutaneous transluminal coronary angioplasty (PTCA)** is when a balloon catheter is passed through a blood vessel to the area where plaque has formed. Inflation of the balloon flattens the plaque against the vessel wall and allows blood to circulate more freely. Also called a *balloon angioplasty*.

- **Venogram**: X-ray film of the veins taken after the injection of dye.

There certainly aren't as many clinical procedures for the lymphatic system, but they are equally important.

Zen and the art of ticker maintenance

Sometimes surgeons have to get down and dirty to fix a heart condition. This typically involves major surgery, a Skilsaw, and lots of time. Though it may be hard to believe that these surgeries are standard issue, remember that heart surgeons perform them every day with great success.

Angioplasty is the surgical repair of a vessel. An *endarterectomy* is an excision within an artery of a thickened interior, usually named for the artery that is being "cleaned out." More vein work includes *phlebotomy*, an incision into a vein to remove or give blood. This is also called *venipuncture*.

The big fun happens when surgeons get more involved with the heart. In *cardiac pacemaker insertion*, a battery-powered or nuclear-powered apparatus is implanted under the skin to regulate the heart rate.

Think bypasses are only for major cities with traffic issues? Not so. The *coronary artery bypass graft (CABG)* is a surgical technique to bring a new blood supply to heart muscles by detouring around blocked arteries, whereas a *femoropopliteal bypass* is surgery to establish an alternate route from the femoral artery to the popliteal artery in the leg, to bypass obstruction.

A *bone marrow biopsy* is just as serious as it sounds. A needle is introduced into the bone marrow cavity, and a small amount of marrow is *aspirated* (removed from the body) and examined under microscope. This procedure is helpful in the diagnosis of blood disorders such as anemia and leukemia.

Also in the category of "beyond serious" is the *bone marrow transplant.* Bone marrow cells from a donor, whose tissue and blood cells match those of the recipient, are infused into a patient with leukemia or aplastic anemia. The patient is first given aggressive chemotherapy to kill all diseased cells and then the donor's marrow is intravenously infused into the patient to repopulate the marrow with normal cells.

Taking a closer look at the lymphatic system's working parts involves the *lymph-angiogram*, when dye is injected into lymph vessels in the foot and an x-ray is taken to show the path of lymph flow as it moves into the chest region. *Lymph-adenography* is an x-ray of the lymph nodes and glands, after the injection of dye.

Terminology Rx: Cardiovascular and Lymphatic Pharmacology

Your friendly neighborhood pharmacist will know all the details of what to use for cardio and lymph-related ailments. In the meantime, you have us. This section lists the most common types of drugs used to correct cardiovascular and lymphatic conditions and diseases.

Antiarrhythmics correct cardiac arrhythmias (irregular heartbeat). Examples include digoxin (Lanoxin) and propranolol hydrochloride (Inderal).

Anticoagulants slow blood clotting. Examples include heparin calcium (Calcilean) and warfarin sodium (Coumadin).

Antihypertensives prevent or control high blood pressure. Examples include nadolol (Corgard), furosemide (Lasix), and diltiazem hydrochloride (Cardizem, Cardizem CD).

Beta blockers treat hypertension, angina, and other abnormal heart rhythms. Metoprolol tartrate (Lopressor) and carteolol hydrochloride (Ocupress, Cartrol) are popular examples.

Calcium channel blockers treat hypertension, angina, and various abnormal heart rhythms. Typical ones are nicardipine hydrochloride (Cardene) and bepridil hydrochloride (Vascor).

Lipid-lowering agents reduce blood lipid (fat) levels, such as niacin (Nicobid), lovastatin (Mevacor), and atorvastatin (Lipitor).

Chapter 17

Just Breathe:
The Respiratory System

· ·

· ·

As you go about your day, you probably don't think to yourself, "Breathe in, now, breathe out," over and over. Perhaps the only time you are conscious of what your respiratory system does is when it is working overtime — during your workout or at the top of stairs you just climbed.

Because the cycle of breathing is continuous and constant, it's easy to take it for granted sometimes. Breathing is something we don't give much thought to as it looks after itself automatically. The body's trillions of cells need oxygen and need to get rid of carbon monoxide, and this exchange of gases is accomplished by the respiratory system.

How the Respiratory System Works

Air contains about 21 percent oxygen that is inhaled through the nose, finds its way to the lungs, into the lungs' air spaces, and passes into tiny capillary blood vessels surrounding the air spaces. At the same time, carbon dioxide — the gas produced when oxygen and food combine in cells — passes from the capillary blood vessels into the air spaces of the lungs to be exhaled. Exhaled air contains about 16 percent oxygen.

External respiration occurs between the outside environment and the capillary blood stream of the lungs, whereas another method of respiration is happening between the body cells and capillary blood vessels that surround them. This process is called *internal* or *cellular respiration*. Internal respiration is the exchange of gases not in the lungs, but in cells of all body organs. Oxygen passes out of the bloodstream and into the tissue cells. At the same time, carbon dioxide passes from the tissue cells into the bloodstream and is carried by the blood back to the lungs to be exhaled.

Capnia comes from the Greek *kapnos*, meaning "smoke." The word now refers to carbon dioxide.

The normal adult cycle of inhaling and exhaling, including a short rest between, takes place about 16–18 times per minute. This is known as the *respiratory rate*.

Figure 17-1 illustrates the respiratory system.

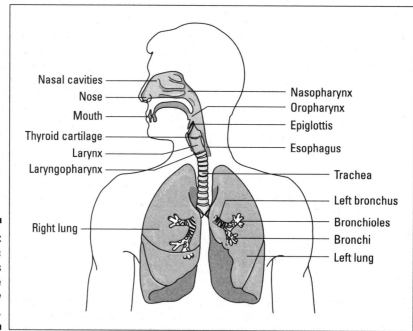

Figure 17-1:
Anatomic
structures
of the
respiratory
system.

Nasal cavities
Nose
Mouth
Thyroid cartilage
Larynx
Laryngopharynx
Right lung

Nasopharynx
Oropharynx
Epiglottis
Esophagus
Trachea
Left bronchus
Bronchioles
Bronchi
Left lung

From LifeARTS®, Super Anatomy 1, ©2002, Lippincott Williams & Wilkins

Nose

When we inhale, or *inspire*, air enters the body through the nose via the external *nasal nares* (nostrils) and passes through the nasal cavity. This cavity is lined with a mucous membrane and fine hairs called *cilia* that filter out foreign bodies (such as dust and pollen) and warm and moisten the air. The *paranasal sinuses* are hollow, air spaces in the skull that join up with the nasal cavity. Paranasal sinuses have a mucous membrane lining and secrete mucus. They make the bones of the skull lighter and help in the production of sound (which is why you sound different when your sinuses are clogged). They connect with the nasal cavity and are named for the bones they are located in: the *frontal, ethmoid, sphenoid,* and *maxillary.*

The singular form of nostrils, or nares, is *naris.*

Pharynx and larynx

After passing through the nasal cavity, air reaches the *pharynx* (the throat), which is made up of three parts. The *nasopharynx* is nearest the nasal cavity and contains the *adenoids*, which are masses of lymphatic tissue, which, in children, if enlarged, can obstruct the airway passage. Below the nasopharynx, closer to the mouth, is the *oropharynx*, where the *tonsils*, two rounded masses of lymphatic tissue, are located. The third part of the pharynx is the *hypopharynx*, where the pharynx serves as a common passageway for food from the mouth and air from the nose. This area is divided into two branches, the *larynx* (voice box) and the *esophagus* (passage to stomach). The larynx leads downward to the trachea, where the air goes down to the lungs. The vocal cords have a slit between them called the *glottis*. Sound is produced as air moves out of the lungs, through the glottis, causing vibration. As food enters from the mouth and air enters from the nose, they both come together in the pharynx.

Adenoid comes from the Greek *aden,* meaning "gland," and *cidos,* meaning "like." The term was once used for the prostate gland. The first adenoid surgery took place in 1868.

What stops food from going into the trachea and respiratory system after it's swallowed? The *epiglottis* is a flap of cartilage attached to the roof of the tongue that acts like a lid over the larynx. When swallowing food, the epiglottis closes off the larynx so that food can't enter.

Trachea

On its way to the lungs, air passes from the larynx to the *trachea* (windpipe), a tube 4 $\frac{1}{2}$ inches long and about 1 inch in diameter. The trachea is kept open by 16–20 rings of cartilage that stiffen the front and sides of the tube. Some of these rings make up the thyroid cartilage forming the projection called the *Adam's apple*.

The Adam's apple is the largest cartilage ring in the larynx. The name is thought to come from the story that Adam sinned when he ate the forbidden fruit and was unable to swallow the apple stuck in his throat.

Bronchi

The trachea divides into two branches called the *bronchi*. Each *bronchus* (the singular form of *bronchi*) goes to a separate lung and subdivides into smaller and finer tubes, like the branches of a tree. The smallest of the bronchial branches are called *bronchioles*. At the end of the bronchioles are clusters of air sacs called *alveoli*. Each *alveolus* (singular of *alveoli*) is made up of a layer of *epithelium*. This very thin wall permits exchange of gases between the alveolus and capillaries that surround and come in close contact with it. The blood that flows through the capillaries takes the oxygen from the alveolus and leaves behind carbon dioxide to be exhaled. The oxygenated blood then carries the oxygen to all parts of the body.

Bronchi comes from Greek *brecho*, meaning "to pour" or "wet." The ancient Greeks believed that the esophagus carried solid food to stomach and the bronchi carried liquids (which it doesn't, and not to the stomach, for sure).

Lungs

Each lung is covered by a membrane called the *pleura*. The outer layer nearest to the ribs is *parietal pleura*. The inner layer closest to the lungs is the *visceral pleura*. The pleura is moistened with a watery fluid that assists in the movement of the lungs in the chest cavity. The two lungs are in the *thoracic* or *chest cavity*. The right lung is slightly larger than the left, divided into three *lobes*. The left lung has two lobes. To remember how many lobes each lung has, remember that the heart resides on the left side of the chest, thus taking up more room and hence leaving room for only two lobes.

One lobe of a lung can be surgically removed without damaging remaining lobes, which continue to function.

The lungs extend from the collarbone to the diaphragm in the chest cavity. The *diaphragm* is the muscular partition that separates the chest/thoracic cavity from the *abdominal* cavity. This muscle aids in the process of breathing. The diaphragm contracts and descends with each inhalation. The downward movement of the muscle enlarges the thoracic cavity area, allowing air to flow into the lungs to equalize pressure. When the lungs are full, the diaphragm relaxes and elevates, making the thoracic cavity smaller, increasing the air pressure in the thorax. Air is then expelled out of the lungs to equalize the pressure. This is called *exhalation* or *expiration*.

Atelectasis, from the Greek *ateles*, means "not perfect." *Ektasis*, "expansion," is an incomplete expansion of the lung, in particular at birth. Incomplete expansion can also occur after surgery when the patient avoids or cannot take deep breaths. This can cause the lungs to remain uninflated long enough for the air sacs to collapse into each other and create dead spaces in the lungs.

Figure 17-2 shows how inhalation and exhalation work.

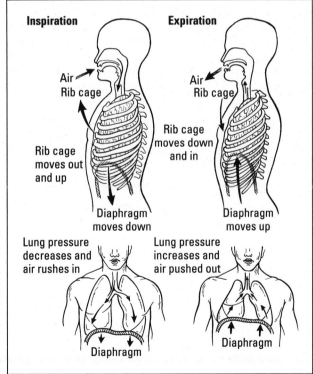

Figure 17-2:
The inspiration (inhalation) and expiration (exhalation) process.

Illustrated by Kathryn Born, M.A.

Short breaths: Respiratory abbreviations

The respiratory system is known for having some, um, long-winded words. Here are some of the more common abbreviations that you can memorize to make communicating about the nose, larynx, pharynx, bronchi, and lungs a little bit easier. You'll be sounding like a cast member of a medical drama in no time.

- **A&P:** Auscultation and percussion

- **ABG:** Arterial blood gases, to determine oxygen and CO_2 levels dissolved into the arteries

- **ARDS:** Adult respiratory distress syndrome caused by injury or illness

- **COPD:** Chronic obstructive pulmonary disease

- **CPR:** Cardiopulmonary resuscitation

- **CXR:** Chest X-ray

- **ENT:** Ears, nose, and throat

- **PFT:** Pulmonary function tests, to determine lung function

- **SOB:** Shortness of breath

- **TB:** Tuberculosis

- **URI:** Upper respiratory infection

- **VPS:** Ventilation perfusion scan, to diagnose pulmonary embolism (also called lung scan or V-Q scan)

Respiratory Root Words

You just got to know about all of the individual parts of the respiratory system. Each one is equally important. The nose without the pharynx or the lungs without the bronchi would be nothing more than spare parts, like on an old junker in a garage. Similarly, the parts of medical terms must coexist and work together to help us understand their meanings. Prefixes, suffixes, and root words work in harmony to bring the world of the respiratory system into focus. Let's start at the beginning, in Table 17-1, with prefixes.

Table 17-1	Start Your Engine with Prefixes
Prefix	*What It Means*
An-, a-	Without, absent
Endo-	Within
Inter-	Between
Intra-	Within

That was simple enough, right? Suffixes outnumber prefixes by more than half, but you should find the list in Table 17-2 still quite manageable.

Table 17-2	Exhale with Respiratory Suffixes
Suffix	*What It Means*
-ar, −ary	Pertaining to
-capnia	Carbon dioxide
-centesis	Surgical puncture with needle to aspirate fluid
-ectasis	Stretching or expansion
-gram	Record
-graphy	Process of recording
-itis	Inflammation
-ostomy	Creation of an artificial opening
-oxia	Oxygen
-pnea	Breathing
-scope	Instrument used to visually examine
-scopy	Visual examination
-stenosis	Narrowing or constricting
-thorax	Chest

Root words and combining forms associated with the respiratory system include the ones listed in Table 17-3.

Table 17-3	Breaking Down Your Respiratory Roots
Suffix	*What It Means*
Adenoid/o	Adenoids
Alveol/o	Alveolus, air sac
Atel/o	Imperfect, incomplete
Bronch/o	Bronchus
Bronchi/o	Bronchial tubes
Epiglott/o	Epiglottis
Laryng/o	Larynx (voice box)
Nas/o, rhin/o	Nose

(continued)

Table 17-3 *(continued)*

Suffix	What It Means
Ox/o, Ox/i	Oxygen
Pharyng/o	Throat
Pleur/o	Pleura
Pneum/o	Lung, air
Pulmon/o	Lung
Py/o	Pus
Spir/o	To breathe
Thorac/o	Chest
Tonsill/o	Tonsils
Trache/o	Trachea (windpipe)

It's All Related: More Anatomical Terms

But that's not all! We still have all sorts of great respiratory words for you to consider. For example, *respirology* is the study of respiratory diseases and respiratory system, and a *respirologist* is a physician specializing in disorders and treatment of respiratory systems.

Getting in and around your body are two gases with which you should be familiar: oxygen and carbon dioxide. Good old *oxygen* is the gas that passes into the bloodstream in the lungs and travels to all body cells. Conversely, carbon dioxide (CO_2) is the gas produced by cells that is exhaled through the lungs. *Internal respiration* is the exchange of gases at the tissue cells. Sometimes, however, these gases are missing. *Acapnia* is the absence or less than normal level of carbon dioxide in blood, whereas *anoxia* is the absence of oxygen in the blood. Some other respiratory-related health issues include

- **Aphonia:** Absence of voice
- **Apnea:** Absence of breathing
- **Bronchospasm:** Sporadic contraction of the bronchi
- **Dysphonia:** Difficulty in speaking
- **Dypsnea:** Difficulty breathing
- **Eupnea:** Normal breathing

- ✔ **Hemoptysis:** Coughing up blood from the lung

- ✔ **Hyperventilation:** Ventilation of lungs beyond normal body needs

- ✔ **Hypoxemia:** Deficient oxygen content in blood

- ✔ **Hypoxia:** Deficient oxygen to body tissue

- ✔ **Mucoid:** Resembling mucus

- ✔ **Mucous:** Pertaining to mucus

- ✔ **Mucus:** Secretion (slime) from the mucous membranes

- ✔ **Orthopnea:** Able to breathe only in upright or sitting position

- ✔ **Nasopharyngeal:** Referring to the nose and throat

- ✔ **Rhinorrhea:** Discharge from the nose

Next we have some terms specifically related to descriptions of respiratory body parts and functions. Get to know the following individual components of the system a bit better:

- ✔ **Adenoids:** A collection of lymph tissue in the nasopharynx

- ✔ **Alveolus:** An air sac in the lung

- ✔ **Apex:** Upper portion of the lung

- ✔ **Apical:** Pertaining to the apex

- ✔ **Base:** The lower portion of the lung

- ✔ **Bronchus:** The branch of the trachea that acts as the passageway into the air spaces of the lung

- ✔ **Bronchioles:** Smallest branches of the bronchi

- ✔ **Bronchodilator:** Agent causing the bronchi to widen or open up

- ✔ **Cilia:** Tiny hairs in the mucous membranes lining the respiratory tract

- ✔ **Hilum:** Middle portion of lung where bronchi, blood vessels, and nerves enter and exit the lungs

- ✔ **Lobes:** Divisions of the lungs. The right lung has three lobes and the left has two

- ✔ **Mediastinum:** Region between lungs in the chest cavity containing heart, aorta, esophagus, and bronchial tubes

Now for the potpourri, the mishmash, and everything but the kitchen sink. Table 17-4 is a grouping of additional vocabulary words that you need to know in order to relate to the respiratory system.

Table 17-4	A Mixed Bag of Respiratory Vocabulary
Word	*What It Means*
Bronchoconstrictor	Agent causing narrowing of the bronchial airways
Bronchodilator	Agent causing widening or clearing of bronchial airways
Hyperventilation	Ventilation of the lungs beyond normal body needs
Mucopurulent	Containing both mucus and pus
Nebulizer	Device creating a fine spray for giving respiratory treatments
Oximeter	Instrument used to measure oxygen in blood
Paroxysm	Periodic or sudden attack
Patent	Open
Pulmonary	Pertaining to the lungs
Rales	Abnormal rattling sounds heard on auscultation
Sputum	Secretion from lungs, bronchi, and trachea coughed up and ejected through the mouth
Ventilator	Mechanical device used to assist with or substitute for breathing when patient cannot breathe unassisted

Common Respiratory Conditions

Of all the most common respiratory conditions, the bronchial tubes get the big daddy: asthma. *Asthma* is attacks of *paroxysmal dyspnea* (wheezing and difficulty breathing) with airway inflammation and wheezing due to contraction of the bronchi, leading to airway obstruction if severe enough. The condition affects millions of people of all ages.

Asthma comes from the Greek *astma*, meaning "to pant."

The lungs have all sorts of wild and wacky conditions associated with them. *Atelectasis*, for example, is the imperfect expansion of air sacs of the lungs. *Emphysema* is the distention of the alveoli with swelling and inflammation of lung tissue. Often seen in heavy smokers, this condition is marked by loss of elasticity of the lungs. *Pneumonia* is the acute inflammation and infection of the alveoli. A couple of different varieties exist: *Lobar pneumonia* involves distribution of infection in one or more lobes of a lung, whereas *pneumocystis carinii pneumonia (PCP)* is an infectious agent caused by P. carinii. It is fungal in origin and is common in AIDS patients.

Pneumonia can be distributed in different ways, for example confining itself to only one lobe, as is often the case with a viral infection, versus presenting a "cotton-wool" appearance on X-ray, with scattered white spots throughout the lungs, as with PCP. It can be caused by many different infectious agents such as viruses, bacteria, and what are known as *atypical agents*, such as *Mycoplasma*, a common cause of pneumonia in teenagers and young adults.

Before 1980, PCP was rare. Sixty to eighty percent of AIDS patients develop PCP.

When we breathe, we don't just breathe in air. Sometimes foreign particles sneak in, like crashers at your respiratory party. Dust is the most common culprit. *Pneumoconiosis* is an abnormal condition of dust in the lungs. Differing types of pneumoconiosis include the following:

- ✔ **Anthracosis:** Coal dust (black lung disease)
- ✔ **Asbestosis:** Asbestos particles in lungs
- ✔ **Silicosis:** Silica dust or glass (grinder's disease)

Speaking of foreign matter hanging out in the lungs, the pleura (that membrane that covers the lungs) can also be affected by foreign matter, namely fluid. *Pleurisy* is an inflammation of the pleura. *Pleural effusion* is the escape of fluid into the pleural cavity. Examples of a pleural effusion include *empyema* (that pus in the pleural cavity you read about earlier) and *Hemothorax*, which is blood in the pleural cavity typically caused by a trauma, is not quite as common but obviously a serious problem — just ask anyone who works in the ER. Other greatest hits of pleural effusion include lung malignancy and congestive heart failure, due to the increased pressure of blood backing up in the pulmonary vessels.

But wait! There's more fluid and pus! It can be a pusapalooza in those lungs, and can often develop into very serious conditions, like these three:

- ✔ **Pulmonary abscess:** Localized area of pus formation in the lungs
- ✔ **Pulmonary edema:** Swelling and fluid in the air sacs and bronchioles, caused by poor blood supply to the heart muscle
- ✔ **Pulmonary embolism:** Floating clot or other material blocking the blood vessels of the lung

If you thought that was all that could possibly affect your breathing, think again. Because there is such a great chance that foreign particles, dust, or communicable disease (from the common cold to more serious conditions), the lungs and its buddies are susceptible to a wide range of conditions. Here are some more examples:

- ✔ **Adenoiditis:** Inflammation of the adenoids

- ✔ **Atelectasis:** Incomplete expansion of the lungs

- ✔ **Bronchiectasis:** Dilatation of the bronchi

- ✔ **Bronchitis:** Inflammation of the bronchi

- ✔ **Laryngitis:** Inflammation of the larynx

- ✔ **Laryngotracheobronchitis:** Croup

- ✔ **Pneumothorax:** Air between the lung and chest wall

- ✔ **Pulmonary neoplasm:** A new growth in the lung, which can be malignant or benign depending on the composition

- ✔ **Rhinitis:** Inflammation of mucous membranes of nose

- ✔ **Tonsillitis:** Inflammation of the tonsils

- ✔ **Tracheitis:** Inflammation of the trachea

Finding the Culprit: Respiratory Diseases and Pathology

Now for the really serious, land-you-in-the-hospital sort of stuff: diseases and pathological disorders. One of the most frightening respiratory diseases is *tuberculosis*, also known as *TB*. Because of its communicable nature, this infectious disease, which is caused by *acid-fast bacilli* spread by inhalation of infected droplets, always causes a commotion when reported to health officials. So much so, in fact, that before antibiotics hospitals built solely for the treatment of TB were quite common. TB is a bit more under control today and is treated with a specific antibiotic regime, usually over a long-term (6-month) period. There are still many cases reported, though, particularly in the Global South.

Diphtheria is another infectious disease of the upper respiratory tract, affecting the throat. *Influenza*, that pesky *flu*, is a highly infectious respiratory disease that is viral in origin. Though for most people nowadays it involves some time off work and chicken soup, the flu can be deadly if not treated, or in high-risk groups like small children and the elderly. *Legionnaires' disease* is a form of *lobar pneumonia* caused by the bacterium Legionella pneumophilia.

Legionnaires' disease gained notoriety after a highly publicized epidemic of it occurred at the American Legion convention in 1976.

Tired yet? Hang in there. There are a few more respiratory diseases you should know. Here's the lowdown:

- **Adult respiratory distress syndrome (ARDS)** is respiratory failure in an adult as a result of disease or injury.

- **Bronchogenic carcinoma** is a cancerous tumor arising from the bronchus. This tumor can *metastasize* (spread) to brain, liver, and other organs.

- **Chronic obstructive pulmonary disease (COPD)** refers to any persistent lung disease that obstructs the bronchial airflow. Examples include asthma, chronic bronchitis, and emphysema.

- **Cor pulmonale** is a serious cardiac disease associated with chronic lung disorders such as emphysema.

- **OSA,** or obstructive sleep apnea, occurs when the pharyngeal collapses during sleep leading to absence of breathing.

- **Pulmonary edema** means fluid accumulation in the alveoli and bronchioles.

- **Pulmonary embolism** is a blood clot, fat clot, or air carried in blood circulation to pulmonary artery where it blocks the artery.

- **URI** is upper respiratory tract infection of pharynx, larynx, and trachea. LRI (lower respiratory infection) usually refers to an infection of everything that's left — bronchi and lungs. It's hard to have a LRI without the URI, but you can have the URI by itself.

Watch those kiddos

Some diseases present in infancy or develop more predominantly in children. One that is commonly associated with children is *pertussis*, more commonly known as *whooping cough*. This is a contagious bacterial infection of the upper respiratory tract (the pharynx, larynx, and trachea). *Croup* (laryngotracheobronchitis) is another respiratory disease affecting children. It is an acute respiratory syndrome in children and infants marked by an obstruction of the larynx, hoarseness, and cough.

On a whole other level are those diseases that can be inherited. *Cystic fibrosis* is one to watch.

This is an inherited disease of infants and children in which there is excess mucus production in the respiratory tract. It is a dysfunction of the exocrine glands with chronic (longstanding) lung disease due to excessive mucus secretion in the respiratory tract, pancreatic deficiency, and sometimes liver cirrhosis. It is a multitude of dysfunctions, but the mucus production is the main problem.

If you are pregnant, consult with your OB about prescreening for cystic fibrosis to determine if you or your partner is a carrier for the disease.

Testing, Testing: Respiratory Radiology and Diagnostic tests

Now that you have all of these conditions and disease terms floating around in your head, you're probably wondering what, if anything, can be done about them? Thanks to the wonders of modern technology, there are all sorts of ways physicians and other medical professionals can diagnose what ails those airways.

To start, physicians rely on their senses to look and listen to what your lungs and associated respiratory parts are doing. Every time, for example, the doctor listens to your heart and lungs with a *stethoscope*, she is performing *auscultation*, which simply means . . . listening to sounds within the body using a stethoscope. This simple method allows doctors and nurses to hear the sounds of the lungs, pleura, heart, and abdomen. Another listening technique is *percussion*, in which the physician makes short, sharp blows (taps) to the surface of the body with a finger or instrument to determine density from sounds of the underlying tissue. A *laryngoscopy* occurs when the larynx is visualized with a laryngoscope. A *bronchoscopy* is the examination of the bronchus by passing a flexible fiberoptic tube (endoscope) into the bronchus. A *tracheostomy* is cutting an opening into the trachea through the neck and inserting a tube to facilitate passage of air or removal of secretions.

IPPA stands for inspection, palpation, percussion, and auscultation. These are all part of a normal physical examination either in hospital or in physician's office.

Diagnostic tests are part of the respiratory physician's problem-solving bag of tricks. Some are more invasive than others, whereas some simply involve more looking and listening with the aid of medical equipment. Some of the most used tests are the following:

- **Bronchial washing:** Specimens can be obtained for bacterial studies and *cytologic* or cell studies, by aspiration of bronchial secretions or by injecting fluid and retrieving it.

- **Endotracheal intubation** is when a tube is placed through the mouth, into the trachea, to establish an airway.

- **Lung biopsy:** Lung tissue is obtained by forceps or brush (bronchial brushing). Can also be accomplished through a catheter inserted under X-ray guidance.

- **Lung scan:** Radioactive material is injected or inhaled and images are recorded of its distribution into lung tissue.

✔ **Pulmonary function tests** evaluate ventilation capacity of the lung. A *spirometer* measures the air taken in and out of the lungs.

✔ **Thoracentesis:** Chest wall is punctured with a needle to obtain fluid from the pleural cavity for diagnostic studies or to relieve pressure in the lung.

✔ **Tuberculin test** is when an antigen is applied to the skin by multiple punctures or tines test, or intradermally by the Mantoux test. An inflammatory reaction is observed in 48–96 hours in an infected patient.

One very useful way to view what is going on in the respiratory system is to use X-ray and endoscopic procedures to take a closer look. Two major types of X-ray are used for this system: A *bronchogram* is an X-ray of the bronchi, and a *chest X-ray* is used to evaluate the lungs and heart. Another widely used diagnostic method is the *bronchoscopy*, a visual examination of the bronchus using a *bronchoscope*. A *chest CT* is also called *computerized axial tomography (CAT scan)*. This is when physicians and radiologists use computerized images of the chest cavity to diagnose tumors, abscesses, and pleural effusion.

Paging Dr. Terminology: Respiratory Surgeries and Procedures

Now you've got the tools to identify and diagnose conditions and diseases of the respiratory system, get your instruments and scrub in, because it's time to operate.

Most of the terms regarding surgeries and procedures revolve around the actual incisions, excisions, and repairs used to treat a myriad of conditions and diseases. As such, these terms are fairly straightforward. You'll see a lot of *-otomy* and *-plasty* suffixes here, denoting the type of procedure.

Start at the top, with repairs made to the nose. *Rhinoplasty* (your standard beak job) is a surgical repair of the nose, while *septoplasty* is the surgical repair of the nasal septum.

Moving down to the throat region, you have the *adenoidectomy*, an excision of adenoids. Similarly, the *tonsillectomy* is an excision of the neighboring tonsils, as well as a sure method of obtaining ice cream.

Two terms relate directly to the larynx. *Laryngectomy* is the excision of larynx, while *laryngoplasty* is the surgical repair of the larynx. Moving on to the trachea, we have the *tracheotomy*, often popularized in television and movies using some non-medical character who must perform one with a bottle of vodka and a Swiss Army knife or ball point pen. But let's leave it to the professionals, shall we? This procedure involves an incision into the trachea. A *tracheoplasty* is a surgical repair of the trachea.

The lungs and chest cavity are next. Here are some of the most common surgeries and procedures pertaining to that area of the respiratory system:

- **Lobectomy:** Excision of a lobe of a lung
- **Pleurocentesis:** Surgical puncture to aspirate fluid from pleural space
- **Pneumonectomy:** Excision of a lung
- **Thoracocentesis:** Surgical puncture to aspirate fluid from the chest cavity
- **Thoracotomy:** Incision into the chest cavity

Terminology RX: Respiratory Pharmacology

Several kinds of medicines are used to treat the respiratory system. Many are used for other systems as well, but they are worth repeating so you will know what is safe to use with direct relation to the lungs. *Bronchodilators* are used to treat asthma, COPD, and exercise-induced bronchospasm. They relax muscles around the bronchi, increasing air flow. They are usually given orally, intravenously, or by nebulizer or aerochamber (inhaler) administered in puffs. *Corticosteroids* are used to control inflammatory responses. *Diuretics* (water pills) are used to treat pulmonary edema.

When you are feeling the effects of a cold or bronchial infection, you probably take one of these next four drug types: *Decongestants* help reduce swelling in mucous membranes of the nose, to relieve stuffiness and allow secretions to drain. *Antihistamines* help dry up secretions. They are effective in treating allergic reactions, but not effective on the common cold. *Antitussives* decrease coughing by suppressing the cough center in the brain. *Expectorants* reduce the thickness of sputum so it can be coughed up more easily. If over-the-counter meds just won't cut it, a prescription may be in order. *Antibiotics* are used to treat respiratory infections, tuberculosis, and pneumonias. *Silver nitrate* can be used to cauterize superficial blood vessels that cause nosebleeds.

Chapter 18

Feeding Time: The Gastrointestinal System

In This Chapter

▶ Finding out how your gastrointestinal system works

▶ Determining root words, prefixes, and suffixes appropriate to this system

▶ Using terminology of the gastrointestinal system to discuss common conditions and diseases

▶ Finding the right terms to use when diagnosing problems

*T*hat big steak dinner leaves you feeling like you need elastic pants for a reason. Your *gastrointestinal* (sometimes abbreviated *GI*) system has to work hard to make all that meat and potatoes into a useful substance that your body can use as energy, and it can only hold so much at one time.

Imagine the local swimming pool at the height of summer. Only so many kids can jump in, because otherwise the water overflows and makes a big mess. It's the same with the gastrointestinal system. If you put too many things in, something's bound to overflow. So, take small bites and try to digest everything there is to know about that full feeling you have after dinner. Elastic pants are optional.

The *gastrointestinal system*, also called the *alimentary* or *digestive tract*, provides a tube-like passage through a maze of organs and body cavities, beginning at the mouth, the food entrance into the body, and ending at the anus, where solid waste material exits the body.

This system and its organs perform three primary functions:

↳ Carrying food for digestion

↳ Preparing it for absorption

↳ Transporting waste products for elimination

How the Gastrointestinal System Works

Digestion begins with our help. Food is put in the mouth. It has to be broken down and digested both mechanically and chemically, as it makes its way through the gastrointestinal tract. Digestive enzymes help speed up the chemical reaction and assist in the breakdown or digestion of complex nutrients from the food.

During the digestive process, proteins break down to *amino acids,* complicated sugars reduce to simple sugars, such as glucose, and large fat molecules are broken down into *fatty acids* and *triglycerides.*

Absorption takes place when the digested food is absorbed into the bloodstream, by going through the walls of the small intestine. By this process, nutrients like sugar and amino acids travel to all cells in the body. Fatty acids and triglycerides are also absorbed through the wall of the small intestine, but enter lymphatic vessels rather than blood vessels.

The third stage is elimination of solid waste materials that cannot be absorbed into the bloodstream. This solid waste, called *feces,* collects in the large bowel and finally exits the body you know where.

You can follow the merry route taken through the various passages and organs that make up the digestive system. Figure 18-1 shows the organs involved.

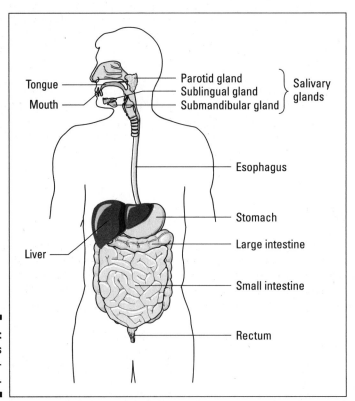

Figure 18-1:
The organs of the digestive system.

From LifeARTS®, Super Anatomy 1, ©2002, Lippincott Williams & Wilkins

Mouth and pharynx

The digestive tract begins with the *oral cavity* or the *mouth*. The lips provide the opening and the cheeks form the walls. The *hard palate* is the roof of the mouth, and the *muscular soft palate* lies behind it, horizontally separating the mouth from the *nasopharynx*, or posterior nasal cavity. Then everything blends in together. The mouth, or *oropharynx*, shades subtly into the *hypopharynx*, or the back of the mouth/top of the throat, and then the pharynx proper, or upper throat, which then becomes the esophagus. And that concludes our discovery tour of the pharynx.

Hanging from the soft palate is a tiny piece of soft tissue called the *uvula*, which means "little grape." The tongue extends from the floor of the mouth and is attached by muscles to the lower jawbone. It moves food around during chewing (*mastication*) and swallowing (*deglutition*). The tongue is covered with tiny projections called *papillae*, which contain taste buds that are sensitive to the chemical nature of foods.

The teeth are important because, during the chewing process, they break down food into smaller pieces to make the swallowing process easier. Around the oral cavity are three pairs of *salivary glands*. These glands produce *saliva*, which contains digestive enzymes. Saliva is released from the *parotid gland*, the *submandibular gland,* and the *sublingual gland*, on each side of the mouth. Narrow salivary ducts carry the saliva into the oral cavity.

Food passes from the mouth to the *pharynx* (throat), a muscular tube lined with mucous membrane. It acts as the passageway for air from the nasal cavity to the *larynx* (voice box) but also as a food passageway going from the mouth to the esophagus. A flap of tissue called the *epiglottis* covers the opening to the larynx and prevents food from going into the *trachea* (windpipe) when swallowing occurs.

Esophagus

The *esophagus* is a 9–10-inch muscular tube from the pharynx to the stomach. It aides in swallowing and propelling the food toward the stomach. *Peristalsis* is the involuntary process of wave-like contractions in the esophagus that helps the food reach its next destination. This process actually takes place throughout the entire gastrointestinal tract, helping to propel food through the system.

Stomach

Food passes from the esophagus into the stomach. The stomach is made up of the *fundus* (top portion), *body* (middle portion), and *antrum* (lower portion). The lining of the stomach consists of folds called *rugae*, which allow the stomach to stretch when food enters. The openings into and from the stomach are controlled by rings of muscles called *sphincters*. The *esophageal* (or *cardiac*) *sphincter* relaxes and contracts moving food from the esophagus into the stomach, and the *pyloric sphincter* allows food to leave the stomach when it has been sufficiently broken down.

The function of the stomach is to prepare food chemically to be received in the small intestine for further digestion and absorption into the bloodstream. Food is churned and mixed with *gastric juices* to make a semiliquid called *chyme*. Food does not enter the bloodstream through the walls of the stomach. The stomach controls passage of food into the first part of the small intestine, so it proceeds only when it is chemically ready and in small amounts.

Liver

The liver, gallbladder, and pancreas are accessory organs of the digestive system. Food doesn't pass through these organs, but each plays a role in the proper digestion and absorption of nutrients.

The *liver* produces greenish fluid called *bile* that contains *cholesterol*, a fat substance, *bile acids*, and several *bile pigments*. Bile is continuously released from the liver and travels down the *hepatic duct* to the *cystic duct*. The cystic duct leads to the *gallbladder,* which stores and concentrates the bile for later use. After meals, the gallbladder contracts, forcing bile into the *common bile duct* joining with the *pancreatic duct*, just before the entrance of the duodenum. The *duodenum* receives a mixture of bile and pancreatic juices.

Pancreas

The *pancreas* produces juices filled with enzymes, *amylase* and *lipase*, to digest food. These pass into the duodenum through the *pancreatic duct*. An endocrine gland (see Chapter 19), the pancreas also secretes *insulin*. This hormone is needed to help regulate levels of glucose in the blood.

The *pancreas* is so named because of its fleshy appearance. Greek *pan* means "all," and *krea* means "flesh."

Gallbladder

The *gallbladder* is a sac-like structure 3–4 inches long tucked under the right lobe of the liver. It is part of the *biliary tract* (hepatic, cystic, and common bile ducts). It stores bile until needed in the duodenum to aid digestion.

You can live without a gallbladder. If inflamed or containing stones (a calcified pebble formed in the gallbladder), it is surgically removed. Bile can find another home in the biliary ducts, allowing the biliary process to function.

Intestines

The *small intestine*, or *small bowel*, extends from the pyloric sphincter to the first part of the large intestine. It is 21 feet long, 1 inch in diameter, and has three parts. The *duodenum*, a foot in length, receives the chyme from the stomach, as well as bile from the liver and gallbladder and pancreatic juices from the pancreas.

Duodenum is from the Latin *duodeni* meaning "twelve each," referring to its length.

Enzymes and bile help digest food before it passes into the second part of the small intestine, the *jejunum*. The jejunum is about 8 feet long and connects to the third portion, the *ileum,* which is 11 feet long. Most of the absorption process takes place in the ileum. In the wall of the small intestine are millions of tiny microscopic *villi*, finger-like projections. Through tiny capillaries in the villi, digested nutrients pass through to enter the bloodstream and lymph vessels. At the lower end of the ileum is the *ileocecal valve*, the joining point of the small intestine to the large intestine.

Here's a quick look at two parts of the intestine. *Jejunum* (Latin *jejunas*) means "empty" and is so named because it was always found empty. *Ileum* (Greek *cilein*) means "to roll." This is a reference to the peristaltic waves that move food.

Excuse me, which is the way out?

If you think a New York City cab driver takes the most indirect route possible, you haven't made the acquaintance of the colon, with its ascending, transverse, and descending sections. That cabbie has nothing on this part of your gastrointestinal system. Obviously named for the direction it takes, this small bowel is very close to the rectum at its most distal end, but it takes the long trip out. It ascends up the right side of the abdomen, transverses across, and then descends down the left side, twisting and turning all over the lower half of your body. Don't even bothering asking for directions!

The *large intestine*, or *large bowel*, extends from the end of the ileum to the anus. It is made up of four parts: the *cecum, colon, sigmoid colon,* and *rectum*. It is five feet long and about 2 $\frac{1}{2}$ inches in diameter. The *cecum* is a pouch that is connected to the ileum by the *ileocecal valve*.

The *appendix* hangs from the cecum. The appendix has no known function, which is why it's not a huge loss to your body if it must be removed. The colon has three divisions: the ascending, transverse, and descending colon. The sigmoid colon is S-shaped, at the end of the descending colon that leads into the *rectum*. The rectum terminates at the lower opening of the gastrointestinal tract at the anus. The entire large intestine receives fluid waste products of digestion that cannot be absorbed into the bloodstream and stores it until it is released from the body.

Gastrointestinal Root Words

A lot of players work together in the gastrointestinal tract. The good news, with regard to word building, is that the list of prefixes and suffixes is a lot less complicated than those of other large systems. The prefixes and suffixes listed in Table 18-1 will help you keep all of the body parts, ailments, and procedures straight.

When in doubt, sound it out!

Table 18-1	Food In, Food Out: Gastro Prefixes and Suffixes
Prefix	**What It Means**
Re-	Back
Retro-	Backward, back

Suffix	*What It Means*
-ase	Enzyme
-flux	Flow
-iasis	Abnormal condition
-lithiasis	Calculus or stone
-lytic	Destruction or breakdown
-pepsia	Digestion
-prandial	Meal
-orrhaphy	Surgical fixation or suturing
-ostomy	Creation of an artificial opening
-tresia	Opening
-tripsy	Crushing

Now, in Table 18-2, it's time to find out what comes in between these word parts. Consider the combining forms and root words as you would the stomach — they break the word down into its most useful component. That root will, in turn, provide the nutritive content that gives the word its meaning.

Table 18-2	The Meaty Part: Gastrointestinal Root Words
Root Word	*What It Means*
An/o	Anus
Appendic/o	Appendix
Bucc/o	Cheek (facial)
Cec/o	Cecum
Celi/o	Belly
Cheiol/o	Saliva
Chol/e, bil/i	Gall, bile
Cholecyst/o	Gallbladder
Choledoch/o	Common bile duct
Col/o, colon/o	Colon
Dent/o, odont/o	Teeth
Duoden/o	Duodenum
Enter/o	Small intestine

(continued)

Table 18-2 *(continued)*

Root Word	What It Means
Esophag/o	Esophagus
Gastr/o	Stomach
Gingiv/o	Gums
Gluc/o, glyc/o	Sugar
Hepat/o	Liver
Ile/o	Ileum
Jejun/o	Jejunum
Labi/o	Lips
Lingu/o, gloss/o	Tongue
Lip/o	Fat, lipids
Or/o	Mouth, oral
Palat/o	Palate
Pancreat/o	Pancreas
Peritone/o	Peritoneum
Pharyng/o	Pharynx
Proct/o	Anus, rectum
Pylor/o	Pylorus
Rect/o	Rectum
Sigmoid/o	Sigmoid colon
Splen/o	Spleen
Submaxill/o	Lower jaw
Tonsill/o	Tonsil
Uvul/o	Uvula

Common Gastrointestinal Conditions

Because the gastrointestinal system is made of many parts, it shouldn't be a surprise that it can be prone to all sorts of ailments and maladies. Mouth conditions are some of the most obvious to the naked eye. Thankfully, two types of professionals can help find solutions to maladies of the mouth that affect mastication (chewing). Ask any parent about your friendly, neighborhood *orthodontist* — she or he specializes in the correction of deformed, crooked, or *maloccluded* (crooked or misaligned) teeth. The *periodontist* specializes in diseases of the tissue around the teeth. Don't forget the good old *dentist*, who takes care of dental issues; and the *oral* and *maxillofacial surgeons* who deal with dental and facial surgery to repair things like cleft palates and dental trauma.

Now, take a closer look at some of the conditions these specialists treat:

- **Aphthous stomatitis:** Canker sores in mouth
- **Bruxism:** Grinding teeth involuntarily, often while sleeping
- **Cleft palate:** Congenital split in the roof of the mouth or upper lip
- **Dental caries:** Cavities in the teeth (*caries* means "decay")
- **Dysphasia:** Difficulty speaking
- **Edentulous:** Without teeth
- **Gingivitis:** Inflammation of gums
- **Halitosis:** Bad breath
- **Herpes simplex:** Cold sore or fever blister on lip or nose due to herpes virus
- **Leukoplakia:** White plaques or patches of mouth mucosa
- **Sublingual:** Under the tongue

Your baby teeth are also called the *primary teeth*. Your first teeth (20 in all) include 8 incisors, 4 cuspids, and 8 molars. Your permanent teeth number 32, with 8 incisors, 8 premolars, and 12 molars.

The esophagus is the next stop on your tour of gastrointestinal conditions. Many of the following conditions result in discomfort both in swallowing (deglutition) and in the digestion process:

- **Aphagia:** Inability to swallow
- **Dysphagia:** Difficulty swallowing
- **Esophageal varices:** Just like varicose veins in the legs; boggy veins with inefficient valves that allow venous backflow, resulting in stagnant blood in bulging veins
- **Esophagitis:** Inflammation of the esophagus
- **Heartburn:** Burning sensation caused by reflux or flowing back of acid from the stomach into esophagus

To keep *dysphasia* and *dysphagia* straight, remember the *s* in dysphasia for "speak," and the *g* in dysphagia for "gag."

Moving south, you find the stomach, an area full of possibility when it comes to conditions. *Gastroenterology* is the study of the stomach and intestines, and a *gastroenterologist* is the physician who treats conditions of stomach and intestine.

Many of the conditions that eventually affect the esophagus or intestine start in the stomach. So, have your antacids ready for these:

- **Dyspepsia:** Difficult digestion
- **Eructation:** Act of belching or raising gas from stomach
- **Gastric ulcer:** Lesion on wall of stomach. Also known as peptic ulcer
- **Gastritis:** Inflammation of the stomach
- **Gastrodynia:** Pain in the stomach
- **Hematemesis:** Vomiting of blood
- **Hiatal hernia:** Protrusion of part of the stomach through the esophageal opening into diaphragm
- **Hyperemesis:** Excessive vomiting
- **Nasogastric:** Pertaining to nose and stomach
- **Nausea:** Urge to vomit
- **Regurgitation:** Return of solids and fluids to mouth from stomach
- **Ulcer:** Sore or lesion of mucous membrane or skin
- **Vomit:** Also known as *emesis*; stomach contents expelled through mouth

The liver, pancreas, and gallbladder all experience their own specific conditions, the most common of which is good, old-fashioned, often-painful *gallstones*.

- **Calculus** (plural is *calculi*): Stones
- **Cholelithiasis:** Condition of having gallstones
- **Duodenal ulcer:** Ulcer in the duodenum
- **Gallstones:** Hard collections of bile that form in gallbladder and bile ducts
- **Hepatomegaly:** Enlargement of liver
- **Hepatoma:** Tumor of liver

All the twists and turns of both the large and small intestines can make for some interesting and often complicated conditions. The sheer length of these organs makes diagnosis and treatment a long and winding road. Start the journey with these intestinal conditions:

- **Ascites:** Abnormal accumulation of fluid in peritoneal cavity caused by cirrhosis, tumors, and infection

- **Borborygmus:** Rumbling, gurgling sound made by move of gas in intestine

- **Cathartic:** Strong laxative

- **Colonic polyposis:** Polyps, small growths protrude from mucous membrane of colon

- **Constipation:** Difficult or delayed defecation caused by low peristalsis movement, over-absorption of water as contents sit too long in the intestine, or by dehydration

- **Diarrhea:** Frequent discharge of liquid stool (feces)

- **Diverticula:** Abnormal side pockets in hollow structure, such as intestine, sigmoid colon, and duodenum

- **Flatus:** Gas expelled through the anus

- **Hemorrhoids:** Swollen or twisted veins either outside or just inside the anus

- **Hernia:** A protrusion of an organ or part through the wall of the cavity that contains it

- **Ileus:** Intestinal obstruction that can be caused by failure of peristalsis following surgery, hernia, tumor, adhesions, and often by peritonitis

- **Inguinal hernia:** A small loop of bowel protruding through a weak place in the inguinal ring, an opening in the lower abdominal wall, which allows blood vessels to pass into the scrotum

- **Intussusception:** Telescoping of the intestine; common in children

- **Laxative:** Medication encouraging movement of feces

- **Melena:** Black stool; feces containing blood

- **Polyposis:** Condition of polyps in the intestinal wall

- **Pruritus ani:** Intense itching of the anal area

- **Steatorrhea:** Excessive fat in feces

- **Volvulus:** Twisting of intestine upon itself

Deadly eating habits

Sadly, some diseases are the result of more serious mental and psychotic disorders, and they can be deadly. If you or someone you know shows any signs of these disorders, please seek medical help immediately. No amount of weight loss is worth losing one's life. Here are the most serious disorders of this type:

✔ **Anorexia:** Psychiatric condition involving self-deprivation of food, lack of appetite, and pathological weight loss

✔ **Anorexia nervosa:** Psychiatric disorder; an abnormal fear of becoming obese

✔ **Bulimia:** Gorging with food and then purging, most commonly by inducing vomiting or use of intense exercise or laxatives/diuretics

✔ **Cachexia:** Generalized poor nutrition (adjective: *cachectic*)

Finding the Culprit: Gastrointestinal Diseases and Pathology

The gastrointestinal system can also play host to even more pathological diseases. Many of these involve inflammation of the various system components, which can cause major disruption to the work the system performs, as well as major discomfort. Here's a look at inflammation-related diseases:

✔ **Cholecystitis:** Inflammation of the gallbladder

✔ **Crohn's disease:** Inflammation and ulceration of the intestinal tract of terminal or end portion of ileum

✔ **Diverticulitis:** Inflammation of diverticula

✔ **Enteritis:** Inflammation of the intestine

✔ **Gastroenteritis:** Inflammation of stomach and intestine

✔ **Hepatitis A:** Acute inflammation of the liver, spread by fecal-oral contact.

✔ **Hepatitis B:** Inflammation of the liver due to a virus transmitted by blood and body fluids

✔ **Hepatitis C:** Virus affecting the liver spread through blood and body fluids. Like other forms of hepatitis, this can cause jaundice, a yellowish discoloration of the skin

✔ **Hepatitis:** Inflammation of the liver caused by virus or damage to the liver

✔ **Pancreatitis:** Inflammation of pancreas

✔ **Periodontal disease:** Inflammation and degeneration of gums, teeth, and surrounding bone

✔ **Ulcerative colitis:** Chronic inflammation of colon with ulcers

As you can see, inflammation is a huge issue with the gastrointestinal system. Here are some other common diseases that can put a halt to this system's daily functions:

✔ **Anal fistula:** This is an abnormal tube-like passageway near the anus communicating with rectum.

✔ **Celiac disease:** Also known as *malabsorption syndrome*, this disease is thought to be precipitated by gluten-containing foods. The hair-like projections (*villi*) degenerate (or actually flatten) so they lose their absorption function. The disease can be hereditary and is common in people of Irish origin. Those with the disease must follow a gluten-free diet to control abdominal pain and diarrhea. Also known as *gluten enteropathy* or *nontropical sprue*.

✔ **Cirrhosis** is a scarring of the liver parenchyma, or tissue, due to damage from alcohol, drugs, and viruses like hepatitis.

✔ **GERD** means *gastroesophageal reflux disease*. It refers to the backward flow of gastrointestinal contents into the esophagus.

✔ **IBS:** *Irritable bowel syndrome* is a group of symptoms including diarrhea, abdominal bloating, cramping, and constipation associated with stress and tension (also known as *spastic colon*).

Testing, Testing: Gastrointestinal Radiology and Diagnostic Tests

Now that you know what can possibly be wrong with your gastrointestinal system, it's time to find out how medical professionals go about confirming their suspicions. There are three primary ways physicians diagnose digestive diseases and conditions: X-rays, ultrasounds, and blood tests. Check out these exciting X-ray methods:

✔ **Abdominal ultrasound:** Most common method to determine the presence of stones in gallbladder, can detect liver cysts, abscesses, gallstones, enlarged pancreas

✔ **Barium enema (lower GI series):** Series of X-rays taken of large intestine after barium enema injected

✔ **Cholangiogram:** X-ray film of bile duct, contrast medium is injected to outline the ducts

✔ **Cholecystogram:** X-ray of the gallbladder

✔ **Upper GI series:** Series of X-rays taken of stomach and duodenum after barium swallow or meal has been taken

Now, don't get squeamish, but it's time to draw blood. That little pinprick you feel when a needle is inserted into skin to draw blood is a small price to pay for all that your doctor can discover just by looking at the results of your blood tests. The blood can tell a million stories about what is going on inside the giant factory that is the body. A wide variety of blood tests can be done to diagnose gastrointestinal conditions and diseases, all of which look for varying levels of enzymes, proteins, and other blood elements. Some of the most common ones are as follows:

✔ **Alkaline phosphatase:** Elevated results indicate liver disease

✔ **Amylase:** Pancreatic enzyme levels elevated in disease of pancreas

✔ **Bilirubin levels:** Present in liver and gallbladder disease

✔ **CBC (Complete blood count):** Measures types and levels of white blood cells (indicators of infection), red blood cells (measures of anemia), and platelets, or clotting factors

✔ **CMP (Complete metabolic profile):** Damaged organs release certain enzymes from their damaged tissue, and these elevated enzyme levels show up in the blood; nonfunctioning organ cannot clean waste products out of the blood the way they're supposed to, and elevated levels of these products also show up in the blood; CMP in particular looks at electrolytes, liver function, and kidney function

✔ **Helicobacter pylori antibody test:** Blood test to determine presence of H. pylori organisms, a bacteria that can be found in stomach lining, causing duodenal ulcer

✔ **Occult blood test:** Test to detect *occult* (hidden) blood in feces; also called *Hema-Check* and *Colo-Rec*

✔ **Protein:** Elevated in liver disease

Some diagnostic procedures are a bit more invasive, such as an *abdominocentesis* (also called *paracentesis*), a surgical puncture to remove fluid from abdominal cavity. Most of the other invasive procedures involve the use of an *endoscope*, an instrument used to visually examine internal organs and body parts. Almost every part of the digestive system can be viewed with the endoscope. The *fiberoptic (all one word) endoscope* has glass fibers in a flexible tube that allows light to be transmitted back to the examiner. The endoscope can be inserted into a body opening (mouth or anus) or through a small skin incision to view internal organs.

Some endoscopic procedures include the following:

- **Colonoscopy:** Visual examination of the colon using an instrument called a *colonoscope*

- **EGD (esophagogastroduodenoscopy):** Visual examination of esophagus, stomach, and duodenum

- **ERCP:** Also known as an *endoscopic retrograde cholangiopancreatography*, this involves an X-ray of bile and pancreatic ducts using contrast medium (like dye) and endoscopy

- **Gastroscopy:** Visual examination of the stomach using an instrument called a gastroscope

- **Laparoscopy:** Visual examination of any internal organ or cavity using an instrument called a *laparoscope*

- **Proctoscopy:** Visual examination of the rectum using an instrument called a *proctoscope*

- **Sigmoidoscopy:** Visual examination of the sigmoid colon using an instrument called a *sigmoidoscope*

Paging Dr. Terminology: Gastrointestinal Surgeries and Procedures

Luckily, many parts of the gastrointestinal system can be repaired using surgical methods such as surgical excision, repair, and suturing. You will likely be familiar with many of these terms, such as *appendectomy*, but some will be brand-spanking new to you. Let's start by taking a look at surgical excisions, or removals. Here are some of the most common:

- **Abdominoperineal resection:** Surgical excision of colon and rectum, by both abdominal and perineal approach

- **Appendectomy:** Surgical excision of appendix

- **Cholecystectomy:** Surgical excision of gallbladder

- **Colectomy:** Surgical excision of the colon or part of the colon

- **Gastrectomy:** Surgical excision of stomach

- **Polypectomy:** Surgical excision of a polyp

- **Uvulectomy:** Surgical excision of uvula

Surgical repairs are next on the to-do list of procedures and surgeries. Gastrointestinal surgical repairs include

- **Anoplasty:** Surgical repair of anus

- **Anastomosis:** Surgical connection between two normally distinct structures

- **Choledocholithotomy:** Incision into common bile duct to remove stone

- **Laparotomy:** Surgical incision into abdomen

- **Palatoplasty:** Surgical repair of palate

- **Pyloroplasty:** Surgical repair of pylorus

- **UPPP (uvulopalatopharyngoplasty):** Surgical repair of uvula, palate, and pharynx to correct obstructive sleep apnea

- **Vagotomy:** Cutting of certain branches of vagus nerve performed during gastric surgery to reduce amount of gastric acid

Finally, surgeons use suturing and the creation of artificial openings to help treat conditions of the gastrointestinal tract. These are some of the most common:

- **Colostomy:** Artificial opening into the colon through abdominal wall

- **Gastrojejunostomy:** Artificial opening between stomach and jejunum

- **Gastrostomy:** Artificial opening into stomach through abdominal wall; this is a feeding method used when swallowing is not possible

- **Herniorrhaphy:** Suture of a hernia to repair

- **Ileostomy:** Creation of artificial opening into ileum through abdominal wall for passage of feces (used for Crohn's disease, ulcerative colitis, or cancer)

- **Jejunostomy:** Creation of artificial opening in the jejunum

Terminology RX: Gastrointestinal Pharmacology

Remember reading that you might need your antacids to get through this chapter? Well, we weren't kidding. *Antacids* are one of the most common and useful over-the-counter remedies for what ails your digestive tract. And most of them provide an added boost of calcium as well. However, keep in mind that over-the-counter (OTC) antacids also have high sodium content, so check with your doctor before using them if you are on a low-sodium diet. Antacids with *simethicone* also relieve excess flatulence, if you need to avoid any embarrassing outbursts in public.

Another great OTC remedy is the *laxative*. This medication relieves constipation. Conversely, *antidiarrheals* relieve or stop diarrhea, and *stool softeners* allow fat and water in the stool to mix in order to soften hard stool.

A doctor may prescribe medications that provide a little more kick, so to speak:

- **Activated charcoal:** Used for its absorption powers; often used via *nasogastric tube* to assist with stomach pumping (drug overdose)

- **Antibiotics:** To treat Helicobacter pylori infections, diverticulosis, ulcerative colitis, and Crohn's exacerbations, and traveler's diarrhea

- **Anticholinergics:** To treat spasms of the GI system such as IBD, divericulitis, and even ulcers; effectively slow down peristalsis with a calming effect

- **Antiemetics:** Control nausea and vomiting. Often prescribed when chemotherapy or radiation is administered

- **Bowel preparations and enemas:** Bowel cleansers taken before barium enema or bowel surgery

- **Emetics:** Used to induce vomiting; especially useful in cases of drug overdose or ingested poisons

- **H2 blockers:** Used to treat gastric ulcers

Chapter 19

Gatekeepers of Health: The Endocrine System

*H*ormones — a word that strikes fear in the heart of even the most manly of men. We're talking the flannel-wearing, beer-drinking, dirt-under-fingernails-even-at-a-wedding kind of guys who run for their lives at the first sign of domestic discord. But fear not, gentle men. It's a frequent misconception that hormones only affect women, but hormones are an important part of every person's physiology. They keep our systems running and send important signals to our major organs that dictate how they work.

Hormones don't just magically appear. They get a little help from their friends, the glands, who are kind enough to produce them, nurture them, and then send the little guys on their way to the appropriate organs.

How the Endocrine System Works

The *endocrine system* maintains the chemical balance of the body. It does this by sending chemical messengers called hormones throughout the body via the bloodstream. *Hormones* regulate and control the activity of specific cells or organs. Slowly released hormones control organs from a distance.

Endocrine glands are located in different parts of the body. They are called *ductless*, because they have no duct system to transport their secretions. Instead, hormones are released directly into the bloodstream. They regulate a variety of the functions of body organs. One can stimulate growth, another matures sex organs, and yet another controls metabolism.

Endocrine: Take *endo*, which means "within" or "inner," and add it to the Greek *krinein*, which means "to separate."

Endocrine glands, no matter which hormone they produce, secrete directly into the bloodstream to the target organ needing that hormone. They are unlike *exocrine glands* — such as the sebaceous glands in the skin — that deliver secretions via ducts directly to the body organ needing them. The endocrine system has two types of endocrine glands: central and peripheral.

The *central glands*, the *pituitary gland* and the *hypothalamus*, are located in the brain. The pituitary gland is referred to as the "master gland" because it produces a variety of hormones that travel via the bloodstream to regulate activities of other endocrine glands. The pituitary and hypothalamus glands work together to regulate body functions such as growth, salt and water balance, reproduction, and metabolism.

Peripheral glands include the *thyroid*, *parathyroids*, *adrenals*, *pineal*, and the *pancreas*. The thyroid, parathyroids, adrenals, and pineal glands have only one function: they produce hormones. The pancreas not only produces hormones but also performs important functions of the digestive system. The pancreas is similar to other mixed function organs, such as the heart, liver, kidneys, ovaries, and testes. In addition to their regular systemic functions, these organs also secrete hormones.

Believe it or not, the heart secretes hormones — as if it doesn't have enough to do already. The heart releases *ANP*, also known as *A-type natriuretic peptide* (or *polypeptide*), which helps to regulate renal and cardiovascular homeostasis. This hormone is released from the heart atria, whereas *BNP* (*B-type natriuretic peptide*) is released from the ventricles. Both help to lower blood pressure.

Figure 19-1 illustrates the endocrine system.

Hormones

Before you get to know the endocrine glands better, take a second to say hello to their little friends, the *hormones*. These little messengers work like diplomatic peacekeepers, so to speak. They communicate with larger organs and systems to maintain chemical harmony and keep your body working. Because the individual parts of the endocrine system produce a variety of hormones, we discuss them in the context of their "home bases" — with each individual gland. Let's look at each of these glands, where they're located, their function, and what hormone they secrete.

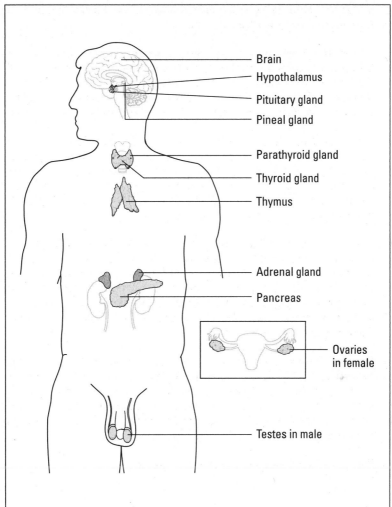

Brain
Hypothalamus
Pituitary gland
Pineal gland
Parathyroid gland
Thyroid gland
Thymus
Adrenal gland
Pancreas
Ovaries in female
Testes in male

Figure 19-1:
The endocrine system.

From LifeARTS®, Super Anatomy 1, ©2002, Lippincott Williams & Wilkins

Pituitary and hypothalamus

The *pituitary gland* — the grand master orchestra leader — is a pea-sized gland consisting of an *anterior* and *posterior lobe*, located at the base of the brain in a small depression of the skull called the *sella turcica*, just below the hypothalamus. The *hypothalamus* secretes *trophic hormones* that stimulate the pituitary gland to release other hormones. Together, these glands are known as central glands.

The *anterior* pituitary secretes seven hormones, messaged by hypothalamus-released hormones. Five of these are trophic (stimulating) hormones that induce other glands to release hormones:

- **The growth hormone (hGH),** also called *somatotropin*, stimulates growth in body cells.

- **The thyroid-stimulating hormone (TSH),** also called *thyrotrophin*, stimulates the thyroid gland to produce and secrete its own hormones, *thyroxine* and *triiodothyronine*.

- **Adrenocorticotropic hormone (ACTH)** stimulates the adrenal cortex to produce and secrete *cortisol* and *aldosterone*.

- **Follicular-stimulating hormone (FSH)** in the female is responsible for the growth of the ovum (egg) in the ovaries and stimulates the secretion of estrogen and progesterone. In the male, FSH promotes sperm (spermatozoa) formation. This is also known as a gonadotropic hormone, one which influences the growth and hormone secretion of the ovaries in females and testes in males.

- **The luteinizing hormone (LH)** induces the secretion of progesterone and triggers ovulation. In the male, LH regulates testosterone secretion. This is also a gonadotropic hormone.

The remaining two hormones do not stimulate production of other hormones, so they are not tropic hormones. *Prolactin (PRL)* is the hormone that promotes the growth of breast tissue and sustains milk production after childbirth. *Melanocyte-stimulating hormone (MSH)* influences the formation of melanin and causes increased pigmentation in the skin.

The posterior lobe of the pituitary gland stores and secretes two hormones. *Antidiuretic hormone (ADH),* also known as vasopressin, prevents excessive loss of water. *Oxytocin* stimulates uterine contractions in childbirth and maintains labor during childbirth. It also regulates the flow of milk from the mammary glands during breastfeeding.

The pineal gland: Endocrine groupie

The pineal gland is a bit of a mystery, a sort of hanger-on to the endocrine system. It is included in the endocrine system because it is ductless. However, little is known about its endocrine function. It is located near the base of the brain and secretes a substance called *melatonin*. This is believed to increase the activity of the reproduction system and regulate the sleep cycle. Calcification of the pineal gland can occur and is used as a radiological marker when X-rays of the brain are examined.

Thyroid

The *thyroid gland* is composed of two pear-shaped lobes separated by a strip of tissue called the *isthmus*. It is located on either side of the trachea, just below a large piece of cartilage called the *thyroid cartilage*. This cartilage covers the larynx and is the prominence on the neck known as the Adam's apple. The thyroid is made up of tiny sacs filled with a jelly-like fluid called *colloid*. The hormones secreted by the thyroid are stored in the colloid until passing into the bloodstream when required.

The thyroid weighs only about one ounce.

The two iodine-rich hormones secreted by the thyroid gland are *thyroxine (T4)* and *triiodothyronine (T3)*. These hormones are synthesized in the thyroid from iodine, which is picked up from the blood circulating through the gland. T3 and T4 are necessary to maintain a normal level of metabolism in the body. Thyroid hormone aids cells in the uptake of oxygen and supports the body's *basal metabolic rate (BMR)*. The BMR is the speed — or lack thereof — at which your body absorbs food, turns it into useful amino acids, fats, and sugars, uses these nutrients, and eliminates the waste. The BMR also refers to your overall energy level, temperature control, skin and hair condition, mood, energy level, and even the rate and effectiveness of your cognitive processes. Injections of thyroid hormone raise the metabolic rate, and removal of the gland diminishes the thyroid hormone content in the body. This results in a lower metabolic rate, heat loss, and poor physical and mental development. The gland also secretes *calcitonin*, which helps maintain the balance of calcium necessary for a variety of processes.

The *parathyroid glands* are four small (about ½-inch) oval bodies that lie on the back aspect of the thyroid gland, two on each side. These glands secrete the *parathyroid hormone (PTH)*. This hormone mobilizes calcium from bones into the bloodstream, where calcium is necessary for proper functioning of body tissue. The adjustment of normal calcium in the food we eat is absorbed from the intestines and carried via the bloodstream to bones for storage.

The adjustment of levels of calcium in the blood is a good example of the way hormones control *homeostasis*, or equilibrium or consistency, of the body's internal environment.

Pancreas

The *pancreas* is located behind the stomach and functions as part of the gastrointestinal system. (We also discuss this gland in Chapter 18.) Consider it a jack of all trades and, as such, a member of more than one body system. As an endocrine gland, the pancreas produces hormones — that is, in this case, specialized cells in the pancreas produce hormones. The cells are called the *islets of Langerhans* and they secrete *insulin* and *glucagon*, both of which play roles in the proper metabolism of sugar and starch in the body. Insulin is necessary in the bloodstream for the use and storage of blood sugar and acts to decrease blood sugar levels, whereas glucagon acts to increase them by instructing the liver to synthesize new glucose in a process called *gluconeogenesis.*

Adrenals

The *adrenal glands* are two small glands, one on top of each kidney. Each gland consists of two parts, an outer portion called the *adrenal cortex* and an inner portion called the *adrenal medulla*. The cortex and medulla are two glands in one, each secreting its own hormone. The cortex secretes hormones called *steroids*, which are complex chemicals derived from cholesterol. The medulla secretes hormones called *catecholamines*, chemicals derived from amino acids.

The adrenal cortex also secretes *mineral corticoids,* also known as *mineralocorticoids*. These hormones regulate the amount of mineral sodium and potassium in the body. The main corticoid, *aldosterone,* is responsible for electrolyte and water balance, affecting blood sodium concentration and potassium. Aldosterone secretion increases in a severe sodium-restricted diet, enabling the body to hold needed salts. *Cortisol*, also called *hydrocortisone*, is a glucocorticoid hormone in that it increases the ability of cells to make new sugar out of fat. The adrenal cortex also secretes *androgens* that aid in the development of secondary male characteristics, such as growth of pubic and facial hair.

Addison's disease, a disease of the adrenal cortex, was named after Thomas Addison, an English pathologist.

Endocrine abbreviations

Some common abbreviations associated with the endocrine system include:

- ✔ **ADA:** American Diabetes Association
- ✔ **BMR:** Basal metabolic rate
- ✔ **DI:** Diabetes insipidus
- ✔ **DM:** Diabetes mellitus
- ✔ **FBS:** Fasting blood sugar

- ✔ **GTT:** Glucose tolerance test
- ✔ **IDDM:** Insulin-dependent diabetes mellitus (more commonly known as Type 1 Diabetes)
- ✔ **NIDDM:** Non-insulin-dependent diabetes mellitus (More commonly known as Type 2 Diabetes)
- ✔ **PRL:** Prolactin

The adrenal medulla secretes two hormones: *epinephrine* or *adrenalin* and *norepinephrine-noradrenalin*. Both hormones work in conjunction with the sympathetic nervous system. Under stress, these hormones are secreted by the adrenal medulla in response to nervous stimulation. They help the body respond to crisis situations by increasing the heart rate, blood pressure, blood glucose (sugar) level, and rate of blood clotting.

Gonads

The *gonads* (ovaries in the female, and testes in the male) are the gamete-producing glands. A *gamete* is a sex cell. Hormones that stimulate the gonads are known as *gonadotropins*.

Estrogen is secreted by the ovaries and is necessary in the development of secondary female sex characteristics (pubic hair and breast development, for example). It also regulates the menstrual cycle.

Progesterone is released in the second half of a menstrual cycle by the *corpus luteum* (empty egg sac) in the ovary. Its function is to prepare the uterus for pregnancy. If fertilization doesn't occur, secretion of progesterone stops, and the menstrual cycle follows. There are small levels of estrogen and progesterone present in males as well.

Human chorionic gonadotropin (HCG) is secreted by the placenta when a pregnancy occurs. This stimulates the ovary to keep producing estrogen and progesterone to maintain the pregnancy.

Testosterone is secreted in the testes. It stimulates the development of secondary male sex characteristics (pubic and facial hair, deepening of voice). The hormone is also present in women to some degree, and some believe it increases female libido.

Endocrine Root Words

The glands of the endocrine system all produce different hormones that help keep the systems of the body running like clockwork. If you consider these glands the gatekeepers of the hormones they produce and send, you can consider prefixes and suffixes the gatekeepers of the root words. They both help tell you more about the meaning of the medical term. Table 19-1 shows some prefixes and suffixes associated with the endocrine system:

Table 19-1	Coming and Going: Endocrine Prefixes and Suffixes
Prefix	**What It Means**
Eu-	Normal
Ex-, exo-	Outside, outward
Hyper -	Excessive, above normal
Hypo-	Below normal
Pan-	All
Suffix	What It Means
-drome	Run, running
-emia	Blood condition
-gen	Producing
-genesis	Production
-ism	Condition

Next, in Table 19-2 we present the nitty-gritty of endocrine terminology. As always, the root words and combining forms let you know more about the condition or location involved with each term.

Table 19-2	Maintaining Balance: Endocrine Root Words
Suffix	**What It Means**
Acr/o	Extremities, height
Adren/o	Adrenal glands
Calc/o	Calcium
Cortic/o	Cortex
Crin/o	To secrete
Dips/o	Thirst
Galact/o	Milk
Gluc/o, glyc/o	Sugar
Gonad/o	Sex glands
Home/o	Sameness or unchanged
Immun/o	Safe
Kal/i	Potassium
Lact/o	Milk

Suffix	What It Means
Natr/o	Sodium
Pancreat/o	Pancreas
Parathyroid/o	Parathyroid gland
Radi/o	Radioactive
Somat/o	Body
Thyr/o thyroid/o	Thyroid gland
Toxic/o	Poison
Ur/o	Urine

It's All Related: More Endocrine Anatomical Terms

It is, without a doubt, incredibly vital that the components of the endocrine system work in harmony because the system is a fairly complex collection of glands that produce a variety of hormones. The specialty study of this system of glands is known as *endocrinology*, with the physician in charge known as an *endocrinologist*.

Here's a closer look at even more aspects of this highly influential system. First, take a look at some hormone-related terms:

- **Adrenalin/epinephrine:** Adrenalin is a traditional trademark for the preparation of epinephrine (adrenaline) in the United States

- **Antidiuretic hormone (ADH):** Hormone secreted to stimulate water reabsorption

- **Cortisol:** Hormone secreted by adrenal cortex

- **Epinephrine:** Hormone produced by adrenal medulla

- **Glucagon:** Hormone produced by pancreas in islets of Langerhans that stimulates the release of sugar

- **Growth hormones (GH and hGH):** Secreted hormones stimulating the growth of long bones; also called somatotropin

- **Hydrocortisone:** Cortisol

- **Insulin:** Hormone secreted by islets of Langerhans; essential for the proper uptake and metabolism of sugar in cells

- **Islets of Langerhans:** Endocrine cells of the pancreas

- **Melatonin:** Hormone secreted by pineal gland
- **Oxytocin:** Hormone secreted to stimulate uterus to contract during labor
- **Renin:** Hormone secreted by kidneys to raise blood pressure
- **Somatotropin:** Growth hormone
- **Steroids:** Complex substance derived from cholesterol of which many hormones are made
- **Target tissue:** Cells towards which the effects of the hormone are directed
- **TSH:** Hormone secretion that stimulates the thyroid gland to produce thyroxine (T3) and triiodothyronine (T4)
- **Vasopressin:** Antidiuretic hormone ADH

Next, take a look at some of the other substances associated with the endocrine system. Though not hormones, these are vital products of this system, and help keep the body functioning properly.

- **Calcium:** Mineral substance necessary for proper functioning of body tissues and bones
- **Electrolytes:** Mineral salt found in blood and tissues; necessary for proper functioning of body cells; potassium, sodium, and calcium are examples of necessary electrolytes
- **Glucose:** Simple sugar
- **Glycogen:** Starch, a storage form of sugar
- **Iodine:** Chemical element composing a large part of thyroxine, produced by the thyroid gland

Protein comes from the Greek *protos*, meaning "first."

Common Endocrine Conditions

Most conditions associated with the endocrine system present more than just a common nuisance or annoyance. These conditions can really mess with the everyday function of your body and its organs. Effects like extreme weight gain or weight loss, extreme height issues, and even *renal (kidney) failure* are not uncommon when it comes to endocrine conditions.

You will notice that many of these common conditions are results of either glandular underactivity or overactivity. Many are also a result of a more serious endocrine disease, such as diabetes, which we cover in the next section.

The following are a list of pathological conditions that pertain to the pituitary gland:

- **Acromegaly:** Enlargement of the extremities due to hyperfunctioning of the pituitary gland after puberty
- **Dwarfism:** Congenital hyposecretion of growth hormone
- **Gigantism:** Hyperfunctioning of the pituitary gland before puberty, resulting in abnormal overgrowth of the body
- **Hypophysitis:** Inflammation of pituitary body
- **Panhypopituitarism:** Generalized insufficiency of pituitary hormones

Moving on to the thyroid, which is not without its own special issues, many of the following conditions involve both size of the gland as well as its output:

- **Cretinism:** Extreme hypothyroidism during infancy and childhood
- **Euthyroid:** Condition of having a normal thyroid
- **Exophthalmos:** Abnormal protrusion of eyeballs
- **Goiter or thyromegaly:** Abnormal enlargement of thyroid
- **Hashimoto's thyroiditis:** A progressive autoimmune *thyroiditis* (lymphocytic invasion of the thyroid gland) with developing goiter; leads to hypothyroidism and sometimes precedes Graves' disease; also called *chronic lymphocytic thyroiditis*
- **Hyperparathyroidism:** Excessive production of the parathyroid hormone
- **Hyperthyroidism:** Overactivity of the thyroid gland
- **Hypoparathyroidism:** Deficient production of parathyroid hormone
- **Hypothyroidism:** Underactivity of the thyroid gland
- **Myxedema:** Advanced hypothyroidism in adulthood
- **Thyroiditis:** Inflammation of the thyroid gland

Exophthalmos comes from the Greek *ex*, meaning "outwards," and *ophthalmos*, meaning "eye." Protrusion of the eyeball can be a symptom of hyperthyroidism, which was originally described by Robert James Graves, an Irish physician. Voilá! We have Graves' disease.

Next is our old friend, the parathyroid, with an odd mix of conditions affecting calcium and, of all things, your wrists. Take a look:

- **Hypercalcemia:** Abnormally high levels of calcium.

- **Hypocalcemia:** Abnormally low levels of calcium.

- **Tetany:** A neurological disorder resulting in spasms (contractions) of a muscle; usually marked by sharp flexion of wrists or ankle joints, most often affects extremities

The adrenals are next on the checklist of conditions. Remember that these glands have one primary function: to produce hormones. So, if these are out of whack, so is your entire body.

- **Adrenal virilism:** Excessive output of adrenal androgens

- **Adrenopathy:** Disease of the adrenals

Now it's time to talk about the pancreas, that double-dipper gland that is involved in the inner workings of more than one system. In the case of the endocrine system, some common conditions can affect the performance of this gland of many talents. They are

- **Acidosis:** Abnormal condition characterized by reduced alkalinity of the blood and of the body tissues

- **Hyperglycemia:** Abnormally high sugar in the blood

- **Hypoglycemia:** Abnormally low sugar in the blood

- **Pancreatitis:** Inflammation of the pancreas

Conditions of the gonads can be troublesome and can cause some problematic side effects, such as heavy or irregular periods and ovarian cysts for women and erectile dysfunction for men. Discussing these conditions, in particular, require a level of sensitivity.

- **Gynecomastia:** Excessive breast development in a male

- **Hypergonadism:** Excessive secretion of hormones by sex glands

- **Hypogonadism:** Deficient secretion of hormones by sex glands

Now, it's time for the potpourri of conditions. Many of these occur as a result of a more serious pathological disease, and some involve too much or too little of a specific substance in your body. It's an endocrine grab bag!

- **Diabetes insipidus:** Insufficient secretion of the antidiuretic hormone vasopressin; causes the kidney *tubules* to fail to reabsorb needed water and salt

- **Diabetic nephropathy:** Destruction of kidneys, causing renal insufficiency requiring hemodialysis or renal transplantation

- ✔ **Homeostasis:** Tendency in an organ to return to equilibrium or constant stable state

- ✔ **Hyperkalemia:** Excessive amounts of potassium in blood

- ✔ **Hyponatremia:** Deficient amount of sodium in the blood

- ✔ **Hyperparathyroidism:** A condition of excess parathyroid hormone secretion, whether from tumor, genetic condition, or medication

- ✔ **Ketoacidosis:** A primary complication of diabetes mellitus; fats are improperly burned leading to an accumulation of ketones in the body

- ✔ **Polyuria:** Excessive urination

- ✔ **Polydipsia:** Excessive thirst

Finding the Culprit: Endocrine Diseases and Pathology

While, admittedly, no condition of the endocrine system is simple or without side effects, the diseases we talk about in this section have especially serious consequences. One of the most common of these diseases is diabetes, which affects millions of people of all ages. Not only does diabetes affect the function of the body, it greatly affects a person's everyday habits. To manage the disease, one typically has to alter the diet and often take medications or insulin injections. Basically, the patient must learn a whole new lifestyle. Read on to find out more about this and other serious endocrine diseases.

The official name of diabetes is *Diabetes mellitus*, which means there is a lack of insulin secretion from the pancreas.

There are two major types of diabetes mellitus:

- ✔ **Type 1 diabetes** is also known as *insulin-dependent diabetes mellitus (IDDM)* or *juvenile* or *child onset diabetes*; it is often seen in children. It involves the destruction of the cells of the islets of Langerhans with complete deficiency of insulin in the body. Daily insulin injections are necessary.

- ✔ **Type 2 diabetes** is also called *non-insulin-dependent diabetes mellitus (NIDDM)* or *adult-onset diabetes*; age and obesity is a common factor. The islets of Langerhans are not destroyed, and there is deficiency of insulin secretion which causes insulin resistance in the body. Treatment includes diet, weight reduction, exercises, and if necessary, insulin or oral hypoglycemic drugs.

Some of the other serious pathological endocrine diseases affect the thyroid and the adrenal glands:

- **Addison's disease** is hypofunctioning of the adrenal cortex. Glucocorticoids are produced in deficient amounts. Hypoglycemia, excretions of large amounts of water and salt, weakness, and weight loss are symptoms of this condition. Treatment consists of daily cortisone administration and intake of salts.

- **Cushing's disease** involves hyperfunctioning of the adrenal cortex with increased glucocorticoid secretions. Hyperplasia of the adrenal cortex results from excessive stimulation of the gland by ACTH. Obesity, moon-like fullness of the face, excessive deposition of fat on the back called "buffalo hump," and high blood pressure are produced by excessive secretions of the adrenal steroid.

- **Thyroid carcinoma** is cancer of the thyroid gland.

Cushing's disease was named after Harvey Cushing, an American neurosurgeon.

President John F. Kennedy had Addison's disease, as did Bev's dog, Barney. JFK and Barney, together forever in the annals of endocrine history.

Testing, Testing: Endocrine Radiology and Diagnostic Tests

That was quite a list of conditions and diseases, no? It would seem that the endocrine system has more potential conditions than Vegas has slot machines. Good thing physicians can use some relatively straightforward tests to evaluate the way the endocrine glands function.

Blood serum tests only require that you to give a few vials of blood at your local lab office. The professionals do the rest from there, running tests that measure the following levels: calcium, cortisol, electrolytes, FSH, hGH, glucose, insulin, parathyroid hormones, T3, T4, testosterone, and TSH. All of these can be evaluated with blood serum tests.

Sometimes all the lab needs is a clean urine sample, so be prepared to pee in a cup. Urine testing can measure the following substances in the urine as indicators of endocrine disease: calcium, catecholamines, free cortisol, electrolytes, ketones, and glucose.

Glucose comes from the Greek *gleukos*, meaning "sweetness."

Some other tests are a bit more complicated, such as the *glucose tolerance test* (GTT), which requires both a blood test and urine sample. This test measures the glucose levels in the blood and urine in specimens taken 30 minutes, 1 hour, 2 hours, and 3 hours after ingestion of 100 g of glucose. The blood test portion measures levels of glucose in the blood, and the urine test measures for ketones in the urine, which is a symptom of uncontrolled diabetes. Other diagnostic tests for the endocrine system include the following:

- ✔ **Estrogen receptor test:** Determines whether hormonal treatment would be useful in cancer treatment by measuring the response of the cancer to estrogen

- ✔ **Goetsch's skin reaction:** Test for hyperthyroidism involving reaction to epinephrine injection, named for Emil Goetsch (1883–1963)

- ✔ **Radioactive iodine uptake:** Thyroid function is evaluated

Some clinical procedures associated with the endocrine system include:

- ✔ **CT scan:** Also known as *computerized tomography* or *CAT scan*, Here transverse views of the pituitary gland and other endocrine organs can diagnose pathological conditions.

- ✔ **Thyroid scan:** In a thyroid scan, a radioactive compound is given and localized in the thyroid gland. The gland is then visualized with the scanner to detect tumors or nodules.

- ✔ **Ultrasound:** Pictures obtained from ultrasound waves can identify pancreatic, adrenal, and thyroid masses. This procedure is also used to diagnose conditions and diseases of many other systems of the body.

Paging Dr. Terminology: Endocrine Surgeries and Procedures

The majority of the surgeries and procedures associated with the endocrine system involve either incision into or removal of a gland. It is important to note in this system that once an endocrine gland is surgically removed, usually for tumor or enlargement, hormone replacement is necessary. Whatever hormone is secreted by the removed gland must be artificially replaced in the body by drug administration.

You should be able to discern what each of the following surgical terms means by looking at the root and the suffix, which either means to remove or to cut (as in an incision). Here's the short list:

- **Adrenalectomy:** Removal of an adrenal gland
- **Hypophysectomy:** Removal of the pituitary gland
- **Pancreatectomy:** Removal of a portion of the pancreas
- **Pancreatotomy:** Incision into the pancreas
- **Parathyroidectomy:** Surgical removal of parathyroid glands
- **Thyroidectomy:** Surgical removal of the thyroid

Terminology RX: Endocrine Pharmacology

Now, let's get to the good stuff — the drugs that can help treat conditions of the endocrine system.

One of the big daddy diseases of the endocrine system is diabetes, which affects millions of Americans. *Insulin* is administered via injection or subcutaneous pump to treat diabetes mellitus type 1. There are several types of insulin, including rapid acting, immediate acting, long acting, and even mixtures of more than one type. *Oral antidiabetics* (hypoglycemic drugs) are used to treat type 2 diabetes.

Thyroid diseases can seriously affect the body's growth, either in a meta or micro sort of way. Sources of drugs and supplements used to treat thyroid disease include desiccated beef or pork thyroid gland. Some are also made of synthetics. *Antithyroid drugs* are used to treat hyperthyroidism. They work by mimicking the thyroid hormone and inhibiting the production of T3 and T4.

Finally, there are drugs used to treat the pituitary gland, most notably *growth hormone therapy* and *hormone replacement therapy.*

Chapter 20

Calming Down: The Nervous System

. . . .

In This Chapter

▶ Finding out how your nervous system works

▶ Determining root words, prefixes, and suffixes appropriate to this system

▶ Using terminology of the nervous system to discuss common conditions and diseases

▶ Finding the right terms to use when diagnosing problems

. . . .

*I*magine that your body is a giant building filled with all sorts of workers. Blood cells, hormones, and all sorts of worker bees run around all day (and night!) making the company work better. At the center of this building is a huge computer system, upon which all the workers great and small depend. The computer is a lot like your nervous system — it's the hard-wiring that controls all of the little activities your body performs. From the voluntary (raising your eyebrows) to the involuntary (the way your eyes dilate), the nervous system helps keep it all humming along better than the newest Mac or PC.

How the Nervous System Works

The nervous system is the body's built-in computer system, but it is far, far more complex than any state-of-the-art computer. With the brain acting as the CPU (central processing unit), messages are relayed via the spinal cord through nerve fibers, providing connections for incoming and outgoing data. The body has more than 10 billion nerve cells whose function is to coordinate its activities. We speak, hear, taste, see, think, move muscles, and our glands secrete hormones, all thanks to the nervous system. We respond to pain, danger, temperature, and touch as well, and we have memory, association, and discrimination. These functions are only a small part of what the nervous system controls.

The nervous system is made up of three subsystems.

- **The central nervous system (CNS)** includes the brain and spinal cord.

- **The peripheral nervous system (PNS)** is composed of cranial nerves that extend from the brain and spinal nerves that extend from the spinal cord.

- **The autonomic nervous system (ANS)** is a division of the peripheral nervous and controls and coordinates the functions of the body's vital organs, such as heartbeat and rate of breathing — functions we don't even think about.

The worker bees of the nervous system are called *neurons*. A neuron is microscopic, but a nerve is macroscopic, that is, it can be seen with the naked eye. A *nerve* consists of a bundle of dendrites and axons. *Dendrites* are the receptive branching fibers of neurons. *Axons* carry impulses away from the cell body. The dendrites and axons travel together like strands of rope.

Figure 20-1 illustrates the nervous system.

The Central Nervous System

The *central nervous system* consists of the brain and spinal cord. The *peripheral nervous system* consists of 12 pairs of cranial nerves and 31 pairs of spinal nerves. The *cranial nerves* carry or transmit impulses between the brain, the head, and the neck. The *spinal nerves* relay messages between spinal cord, the chest, abdomen, and the extremities. The functions of the spinal and cranial nerves are mainly voluntary, involving smell, taste, sight, hearing, and muscle movement.

Brain

The *brain* is the central control center for regulating and coordinating body functions. It lies in the *cranial cavity* (within the skull). The *spinal cord*, continuous with the lower part of the brain, passes through the *foramen magnum*, an opening in the skull that allows the spinal cord to continue down through the vertebral column.

Most brains weigh between 2.5–4 pounds (40–60 ounces). The size of the skull offers only a general idea of the brain size, because the shape and thickness of the skull varies.

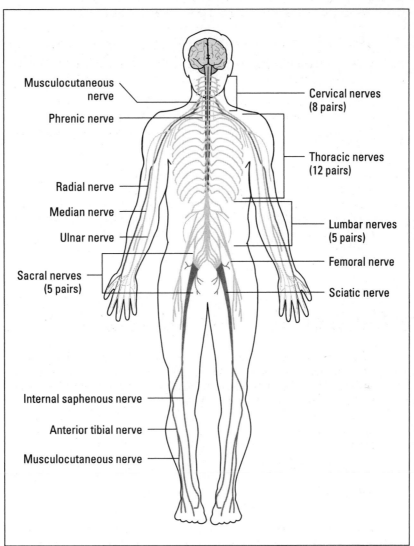

Musculocutaneous nerve

Phrenic nerve

Radial nerve

Median nerve

Ulnar nerve

Sacral nerves (5 pairs)

Cervical nerves (8 pairs)

Thoracic nerves (12 pairs)

Lumbar nerves (5 pairs)

Femoral nerve

Sciatic nerve

Internal saphenous nerve

Anterior tibial nerve

Musculocutaneous nerve

Figure 20-1:
The nervous
system.

From LifeARTS®, Super Anatomy 1, ©2002, Lippincott Williams & Wilkins

The brain's largest part is the *cerebrum*. Nervous tissue covering the cerebrum is called the *cerebral cortex*. The cortex is arranged in folds called *gyri* and depressions or grooves known as *fissures* or *sulci*.

Cerebral hemispheres are the paired right and left halves of the cerebrum that occupy most of the brain cavity. The left cerebral hemisphere controls the right side of the body, and the right hemisphere controls the left side.

Thought, memory, judgment, and association all take place in the cerebrum. *Efferent cranial nerves* carry motor impulses from the cerebrum to muscles and glands to produce movement and activity. The outer surface of the cerebrum, the *cerebral cortex*, is made up of gray matter, and underneath this the *white matter* forms the central part of the brain.

The cerebral cortex is the center that controls speech, vision, smell, movement, hearing, and thought processes and has four *lobes*:

- ✔ **The frontal lobe** is the center for voluntary movement, judgment, reasoning, and impulse inhibition.

- ✔ **The occipital lobe** (the back of each of the hemispheres) manages visual perception, association, and visual memory.

- ✔ **The parietal lobe** collects, recognizes, and organizes sensations of pain, touch, movement, and position.

- ✔ **The temporal lobe** correlates auditory and visual memory as well as language development.

In the middle of the cerebrum are spaces called *ventricles*. These spaces contain watery fluid that flows through the brain and around the spinal cord, called the *cerebrospinal fluid (CSF)*. It protects the brain and spinal cord from shock, acting like a cushion. CSF can be withdrawn for diagnostic purposes or for relief of pressure on the brain.

The *cerebellum*, sometimes called the *hindbrain* because it is located under the back portion of the cerebrum, functions to assist in the coordination of voluntary body movement and maintaining body balance. The *brainstem* is a stem-like portion of the brain that connects the brain to the spinal cord. The *pons*, meaning "bridge," connects the cerebrum with the cerebellum and the brainstem. The *thalamus* acts as a relay station for body sensations such as pain, and the *hypothalamus* controls body temperature, sleep, appetite, and the pituitary gland.

The *medulla oblongata*, located between the pons and the spinal cord, regulates the centers that control respiration, heart rate, blood vessels, and the respiratory system. This is also sometimes known as the *reptilian brain*. It is the last part of the brain to shut down at death.

Spinal cord

The *spinal cord* passes through the vertebral canal from the medulla oblon-gata to the second *lumbar vertebra*. The spinal cord conducts nerve impulses to and from the brain. The cord carries all nerves that affect limbs and lower body and is a passageway for impulses getting to and from the brain.

A cross-section of the spinal cord shows an inner section of gray matter that contains cell bodies and dendrites of peripheral nerves, and an outer region of white matter that contains nerve fiber, surrounded by *myelin* sheaths, con-ducting impulses to and from the brain.

Meninges are three layers of connective tissue membrane surrounding the brain and spinal cord. The outer membrane, the *dura mater*, is a thick, tough membrane containing channels for blood to come into the brain tissue. The second layer around the brain and spinal cord, the *arachnoid membrane* (*arachnoid* meaning "spider-like"), is loosely attached to other meninges. The *subdural space* is a potential space between the dura mater and the arachnoid that contains blood vessels. A space between the fibers and the third mem-brane is called the *subarachnoid space,* and it contains the *cerebrospinal fluid.* A third layer of meninges, closest to the brain and spinal cord, called the *pia mater,* is made up of delicate connective tissue with a rich supply of blood vessels.

The Latin translation of *dura mater* means "hard mother," whereas *pia mater* means "soft mother." *Meninges* were first named by a Persian doctor in the 10th century. When translated into Latin, that changes to *dura mater. Mater* was used because Persians thought that meninges were the mother of all other body membranes.

Peripheral Nervous System

It's worth mentioning here that the nervous system is one giant system that is subdivided into the central nervous system (which we just covered) and the peripheral nervous system. The peripheral nervous system then divides into two parts: the somatic system and the autonomic system. The auto-nomic system further divides to include sympathetic and parasympathetic systems. All subdivisions connect in some way to perform their functions, but they all remain part of the main nervous system.

The peripheral nervous system consists of the somatic system, or voluntary nervous system, whose actions we consciously control. Then there are groups of nerves that function involuntarily or automatically, without conscious control. These nerves compose the *autonomic nervous system*. This is system made up of nerve fibers and carries impulses from the central nervous system to glands, the heart, blood vessels, and the involuntary muscles, such as those found in the walls of the intestines and hollow organs — the stomach and urinary bladder, for example.

Peripheral nerves have different names, depending on the direction of the impulse they carry. *Afferent nerves* carry impulses to the brain and spinal cord from receptors like the skin, eyes, ears, and nose. *Efferent nerves* carry impulses from the central nervous system to organs that produce a response.

The automatic nervous system is further divided into the *sympathetic* and *parasympathetic systems*. Some of the autonomic nerves are called *sympathetic nerves*. The sympathetic nerves stimulate the body in times of stress and crisis by increasing the heart rate, dilating airways to supply more oxygen, and increasing blood pressure. Conversely, the parasympathetic nerves relax the involuntary nerves to calm you down.

Nervous Root Words

Now you know the major players in the nervous system. It's hard to believe the brain and spinal cord hold so much responsibility for the way your entire body functions. And like a supercomputer, one small glitch in how the neurons fire or how the messages are sent down the spinal cord can make the difference between, say, walking and being confined to a wheelchair.

Now let's start building some vocabulary. Table 20-1 lists prefixes and suffixes associated with the nervous system.

Table 20-1   Relax with Nervous Prefixes and Suffixes

Prefix	What It Means
Hemi-	Half
Para-	Beyond, around, beside
Polio-	Gray
Quadri-	Four
Sub-	Below, under
Suffix	What It Means
-algia	Pain
-itis	Inflammation

Prefix	What It Means
-malacia	Softening
-paresis	Slight paralysis
-plegia	Paralysis
-schisis	Cleft or splitting
-thenia	Lack of strength
-us	Condition

Table 20-2 lists nervous root words and combining forms.

Table 20-2	Nerve-Wracking Root Words
Root Word	What It Means
Algesi/o	Excessive sensitivity to pain
Cerebell/o	Cerebellum
Cerebr/o	Brain, cerebrum
Dur/o	Dura mater
Ech/o	Sound
Encephal/o	Brain
Esthesi/o	Feeling, nervous, sensation
Gli/o	Glue
Kinesi/o	Movement
Mening/o	Membrane
Meningi/o	Meninges
Ment/o, phren/o	Mind
Myel/o	Spinal cord
My/o	Muscle
Neur/o	Nerve
Phas/o	Speech
Psych/o	Mind
Thalam/o	Thalamus
Ventricul/o	Ventricle

It's All Related: More Nerve-Wracking Terms

So, here it is: The potpourri, the mish-mash, the great melting pot of nervous system terms. These are some of the most common phrases you'll hear in the doctor's office and hospital:

- **Anesthesia:** Without or loss of feeling or sensation

- **Anesthesiologist:** Physician who administers an *anesthetic* (a drug that reduces feeling)

- **Ataxia:** Lack of muscle coordination

- **Coma:** State of profound unconsciousness

- **Convulsion:** Sudden involuntary contractions of a group of muscles

- **Dementia:** Mental decline

- **Disorientation:** A state of confusion as to time, place, or identity

- **Gait:** A matter or style of walking

- **Monoplegia:** Paralysis of one limb

- **Neurologist:** Physician who specializes in *neurology*, the scientific study of the nervous system

- **Neurology:** The branch of medicine dealing with the study of the nervous system, functions and disorders

- **Paraplegia:** Paralysis of the lower half of the body

- **Postictal:** Occurring after a seizure or attack

- **Psychiatrist:** Physician who treats mental disorders

- **Psychiatry:** Branch of medicine that deals with treatment of mental disorders (disorders without any identifiable pathological cause)

- **Psychogenic:** Produced or caused by psychological factors

- **Psychogenetic:** Originating in the mind

- **Psychologist:** Specialist in psychology

- **Psychology:** The study of the mind, mental processes, and behavior

- **Psychosomatic:** Pertaining to the mind and the body

- **Quadriplegia:** Paralysis of all four limbs

- **Seizure:** Sudden involuntary contractions (convulsion)

Common Nervous Conditions

Because the nervous system is involved in so many aspects of your body's function, the conditions that affect it can have long-lasting implications on all bodily systems. Let's take a look at some of the pathological conditions pertaining to the central nervous system:

- **Aphasia** involves loss or impairment of the ability to speak.

- **Cerebrovascular accident (CVA)** is also known as a *stroke*. It can be a rupture (*hemorrhagic stroke*) or obstruction of an artery (*ischemic stroke*), producing headache, nausea, vomiting, possible coma, paralysis, and aphasia.

- **Coma** is a state of unconsciousness in which a person cannot be aroused.

- **Concussion** is a temporary dysfunction after injury, usually clearing within 24 hours. It's basically a bruise on the brain.

- **Dysphasia** is the condition of having difficulty speaking.

- **Epilepsy** refers to a sudden disturbance of the nervous system functioning due to abnormal electrical activity of the brain. It can manifest by a *grand mal seizure*, with loss of consciousness, limb contractions, and incontinence. It could also be as minor as an *absence seizure*, in which the person appears be "spaced out" for a moment.

  The Greek *epilepsia* means "seizure" and is derived from *epi* meaning "upon" and *lambancia* meaning "to seize." Officially, the term means "seized upon."

  Grand mal (large) seizures (also called *tonic-clonic* seizures) are characterized by severe convulsions and unconsciousness. *Petit mal* (small) seizures (also called *absence seizures*) consist of momentary lapses of consciousness.

- **Hemiparesis** is slight paralysis of half (either right or left side) of the body.

- **Hemiplegia** is paralysis of the right or left side of body often occurring after a stroke.

- **Hydrocephalus** refers to an abnormal accumulation of fluid in the ventricles of the brain.

- **Irreversible coma** is a coma from which there is no response to stimuli, no spontaneous movement, and a flat or inactive *electroencephalogram* (a record of the brain's activity). This is what is known as a brain death.

- **Meningocele** is the protrusion of the meninges through a defect in the skull or vertebral column.

- **Myasthenia gravis** is muscle weakness marked by progressive paralysis that can affect any muscle in the body, but mainly those of the face, tongue, throat, and neck.

- **Neuralgia** means pain in a nerve.

- **Neuritis** is inflammation of a nerve.

- **Neuroma** is a tumor made up of nerve cells.

- **Neurosis** is an emotional disorder involving an ineffective way of coping with anxiety.

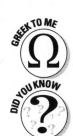

- **Palsy** means paralysis. One of the most common examples is *cerebral palsy*, a partial paralysis and lack of muscle coordination due to damage to the cerebrum of a fetus during pregnancy.

  Paraplegia: The Greek *para* means "beside," and *plegia* means "paralysis."

  Bell's palsy involves facial paralysis due to a disorder of the facial nerve; the cause is unknown, but complete recovery is possible.

- **Polyneuritis** is the inflammation of many nerves.

- **Psychosis** refers to a major mental disorder characterized by extreme derangement, often accompanied by delusions and hallucinations.

- **Shingles**, also known as *herpes zoster,* is a viral disease affecting peripheral nerves. Blisters and pain spread in a band-like pattern following the route of peripheral nerves affected.

- **Subdural hematoma** is a blood tumor below the dura mater, produced by the collection of blood in tissue or a cavity.

- **Syncope** means fainting or sudden loss of consciousness.

Finding the Culprit: Nervous Diseases and Pathology

The diseases and more serious pathological conditions of the nervous system, again, have major implications for the way the rest of your body functions. From the way your muscles move to the coordination of involuntary reflexes, your nervous system can be subject to a wide range of serious pathological issues. Here are just a few of them:

✔ **Alzheimer's disease:** Brain disorder marked by deterioration in mental capacity, caused by atrophy (wasting away) of the brain cells; develops gradually; early signs are loss of memory for recent events, and an impairment of judgment and comprehension

✔ **Amyotrophic lateral sclerosis (ALS):** Also called *Lou Gehrig disease*, a progressive muscular atrophy or wasting away, caused by hardening of nerve tissue in the spinal cord

✔ **Meningitis:** Inflammation of the meninges caused by bacteria (*bacterial meningitis*) or a virus (*viral meningitis*), an infection of subarachnoid spaces

✔ **Multiple sclerosis (MS):** Destruction of the myelin sheath around nerve fibers; scar tissue forms and prevents the conduction of nerve impulses causing muscle weakness and paralysis

✔ **Parkinson's disease:** Degeneration of the nerves of the brain, occurring in later life, leading to tremors, weakness of muscles, and slowness of movement; a progressive condition that leads to muscle stiffness, shuffling gait (manner of walking), and forward-leaning posture

Dr. James Parkinson, an English physician, described Parkinson's disease in 1817. It is also called *parkinsonism, paralysis agitans,* and *shaking palsy.*

✔ **Reye's syndrome:** Disease of the brain and other organs, such as the liver; affects children in adolescence; cause unknown but typically follows a viral infection

✔ **Spina bifida:** Congenital defect of the spinal column due to malunion of the vertebral parts

✔ **Spina bifida occulta:** Vertebral lesion covered with skin and not seen; evident only on x-ray examination

✔ **Transient ischemic attack (TIA):** Sudden deficient supply of blood to the brain lasting a short time; sometimes called a "baby" stroke

Testing, Testing: Nervous Radiology and Diagnostic Tests

Now that you've read about some of the nervous system's conditions and diseases, here's a bit about how to diagnose them. Because many of the following tests deal with delicate parts, such as the spinal cord and brain, physicians try to keep invasive measures to a minimum. It's certainly a good idea to find a solid, reputable facility you feel comfortable with instead of going to Joe Bob's House of MRIs.

Tumors: Unwelcome guests

Tumors are another serious pathological issue affecting the nervous system. Working much the way a virus attacks a computer, tumors attach, grow, and wreak general havoc on anything they touch.

A *glioma* occurs in the brain tissue, whereas a *meningioma* arises from the meninges. Gliomas are highly malignant tumors that almost never metastasize or spread. Example of a glioma is an *astrocytoma*, a tumor composed of *astrocytes*. Gliomas are usually removed surgically. Meningiomas are most often benign and surrounded by a capsule, but may cause compression or distortion on the brain.

Another type of tumor is a *neuroblastoma*. This is a malignant tumor arising from nerve cells. It may be inherited and occurs most often in adrenal glands; it occurs in childhood and is treated with combined surgery and chemotherapy.

And now, to the testing:

- ✔ **Cerebral angiography:** *Contrast medium* (such as dye) is injected into an artery, and X-rays are taken of the blood vessel systems of the brain. This is also called *arteriography*.

- ✔ **Cerebrospinal fluid analysis** analyzes cell count, bacterial smears, and cultures of the CSF when disease of the meninges or the brain is suspected.

- ✔ **Computerized tomography (CT) scans** are performed on the brain to locate a tumor, foreign matter, or blocked vessel.

- ✔ **Electroencephalography (EEG)** is a recording of the electrical activity of the brain, performed to diagnose epilepsy.

- ✔ **Lumbar or spinal puncture** is when cerebrospinal fluid is withdrawn for analysis from between two lumbar vertebrae. Contrast medium for X-ray studies such as a *myelogram* or *intrathecal medicine* may be administered via lumbar puncture procedure.

- ✔ **Magnetic resonance imaging (MRI)** is a noninvasive technique producing cross-sectional and vertical images of soft tissues of the brain by use of magnetic waves. Unlike a CT scan, the MRI produces images without the use of radiation or contrast medium. It is used to visualize tumors, edema, and to confirm multiple sclerosis.

- ✔ **Myelogam** is a procedure in which contrast medium is injected into the CSF, and X-rays are taken of the spinal cord.

- ✔ **Positron emission tomography (PET)** is a technique that permits viewing of a slice of the brain and gives information of brain function such as blood flow.

Paging Dr. Terminology: Nervous Surgeries and Procedures

Most surgeries of this system involve removal of tumors in the brain itself, whether malignant or benign. Tumors of the spinal cord can also be removed surgically. Surgery on the brain and the spinal cord is, as you might imagine, *very* involved and detailed, due to the complexity of nerves and the tissue involved. So, again, think reputable institution and not Craniotomy Mart.

But, we digress. Let's start getting inside your head, literally:

- **Craniotomy:** Surgical cutting into and opening the skull to gain access to the brain tissue for surgery
- **Laminectomy:** Excision of the posterior arch of a vertebra
- **Neurectomy:** Excision of a nerve
- **Neuroplasty:** Surgical repair of a nerve

Terminology RX: Nervous Pharmacology

Now it's time to treat yourself to some drugs. Here are some common types of medications used to treat disorders and conditions of the nervous system:

- **Anticonvulsants, hypnotics, and sedatives** are used to treat various types of seizures.
- **CNS stimulants** are used to treat attention deficit disorders.
- **Cognition adjuvant therapy** is given to treat Alzheimer's disease.
- **Hypnotics** are used to treat sleeping disorders; examples include barbiturates and nonbarbiturates.

The Greek root of *hyponotics*, *hypos*, means "to sleep."

Part V
Name That Plumbing

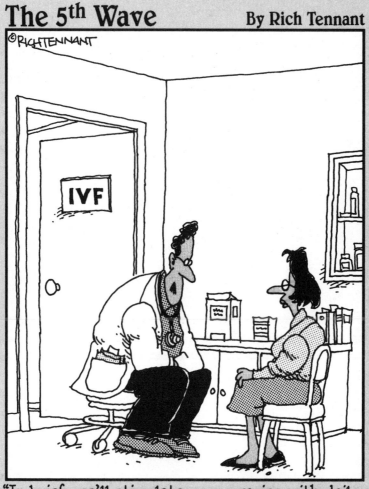

©RICHTENNANT

IVF

"In brief, we'll stimulate your ovaries with daily medications or hormones, perform an oocyte retrieval at the hospital, incubate the eggs in a petri dish at the laboratory, and then sit back and let nature take its course."

In this part . . .

The urinary and reproductive systems are so vital to our way of living and maintaining life that they get their own part, short though it may be. Chapter 21 covers everything you ever needed to know about how your body makes pee. Chapters 22 and 23, respectively, go into details about the male and female reproductive systems, answering the age old question, "Mommy, where do babies come from?"

Chapter 21

When You Gotta Go: The Urinary System

. . . .

In This Chapter

▶ Figuring out how your urinary system works

▶ Checking out root words, prefixes, and suffixes appropriate to this system

▶ Using terminology of the urinary system to discuss common conditions and diseases

▶ Finding the right terms to use when diagnosing problems

. . . .

*Y*ou probably don't give much thought to how your urinary plumbing works every time you use the restroom. However, it becomes a major concern the minute your, uh, output, isn't putting out like it should. Welcome to the wonderful world of the urinary system! From kidneys to bladders, your body is full of all sorts of parts whose sole purpose is to clean your system of toxins by way of creating urine.

Believe it or not, a whole arm of the medical profession is dedicated to helping you add your contribution to the toilet bowl on a regular basis. So the next time you see someone with a license plate that reads, for example, 2PCME, you can bet it's a urologist on the way to work, to be a human plumber of sorts. Let's take a look at what takes up so much of his or her time.

How the Urinary System Works

The urinary system is made up of the *kidneys* (you have two), *ureters* (also two), *bladder*, and *urethra* (one). This system's main function is to remove urea, the waste product of metabolism, from the bloodstream and excrete the urea (in the urine) from the body.

So, how does that big steak dinner you ate last night turn into the next morning's output in the form of urine? Well, food and oxygen combine in cells to produce energy, a process called *catabolism*. In the process, food and oxygen are not destroyed, but small particles making up the food and oxygen are rearranged in new combinations, and part of the result is waste products. Waste products in the form of gases (carbon dioxide) are removed from the body by exhaling through the lungs. *Nitrogenous* waste (the by-product of protein food) is more difficult to excrete from the body than gases. This kind of waste is secreted as a soluble dissolved in water, a waste substance called urine. The main function of the urinary system is to remove urea from the bloodstream.

Urea is formed in the liver from *ammonia* (which is, believe it or not, basically the same stuff you use to clean the kitchen). The bloodstream carries it (in the same manner as hormones and lymph) to the kidneys, where it passes with water, salts, and acids out of the bloodstream into the kidneys. The kidneys remove waste products, producing urine that travels through each ureter into the bladder. Urine is then excreted from the bladder via the urethra. Magically (or so it might seem), your steak dinner has turned into pee!

Figure 21-1 shows the urinary system.

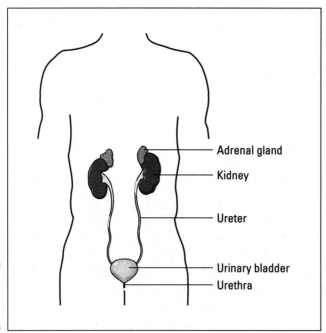

Figure 21-1:
The urinary
system.

- Adrenal gland
- Kidney
- Ureter
- Urinary bladder
- Urethra

From LifeARTS®, Super Anatomy 1, ©2002, Lippincott Williams & Wilkins

Kidneys

You have two *kidneys*, unless you've had one removed. Kidneys are dark reddish brown, bean-shaped organs that are located behind the abdominal cavity on each side of the spine in the lumbar region. They are embedded in a cushion of *adipose* (fat) tissue and surrounded by connective tissue for support. Each kidney is about the size of a fist and weighs approximately 8 ounces. The left kidney is a little larger and sits a little higher than the right one.

Each kidney consists of an outer *cortex* and an inner *medulla* region. The cortex contains millions of nephrons, and the medulla contains the collecting *tubules* (small tubes). A segment on the medial border of each kidney, called the *hilum*, allows the blood vessels, nerves, and ureter to pass through. The *nephron* is the kidney's functional and structural unit, or the "brains" of the kidney. Each is a urine-producing microscopic structure, consisting of a *renal corpuscle* and *renal tubule*.

Hilum's Latin meaning is "a small thing or a trifle." This is a term for a depression or pit in an organ where vessels and nerves enter.

Glomeruli (singular *glomerulus*) are clusters of *capillaries* (small vessels) at the entrance of each nephron. They help filter the blood, beginning the process of urine production. In the blood-filtering process, water and solutes from the blood in the glomeruli pass through the capillaries and the walls that make up the glomeruli into the tubules. Tubules have the ability to remove substances your body needs and return them to the blood.

The Greek word *pyelos* means "tub-shaped vessel," which describes the shape of each kidney.

The story behind what's in the bowl

Here are the vital stats of your wee-wee. Normal urine is translucent pale amber in color with the distinctive odor you are familiar with. It consists of 95 percent water with dissolved substances, nitrogenous waste, pigments, toxins, hormones, and sometimes abnormal substances like blood, glucose (sugar), and albumin. Of course, if your naked eye can see blood in your urine, it's time to call your physician.

Average urine output in a 24-hour period is approximately 1000–2000 mL (milliliters). Urine's normal *specific gravity* should be somewhere between 1.015 and 1.025. Specific gravity is the weight of a substance compared with the weight of some other substance taken as a standard. Water is the usual standard in liquids. The specific gravity of water is 1. If urine shows a specific gravity of 1.025, it means the urine is 1.025 times heavier than water.

Be on the lookout for dark yellow urine. This means your pee is overly concentrated, which may indicate a degree of dehydration.

Ureters

You have two *ureters* (right and left). They are muscular tubes about 15–18 inches long, lined with mucous membrane, extending from the renal pelvis down to the bladder. The left ureter is longer because the left kidney sits higher in position. The urine enters the bladder in spurts via each ureter every 10–30 seconds.

At the bladder entrance is a *ureteral orifice* (opening) that opens to allow urine into the bladder from each ureter. The orifice works in sequence with the *peristaltic* (wave-like) action that propels the urine through the ureter. This action prevents urine from flowing back into the ureter when the bladder contracts.

Urinary bladder

The *urinary bladder* is a hollow, very elastic muscular sac in the pelvic cavity. It acts as a temporary reservoir or "holding tank" for urine. It has two openings to receive the urine coming from each ureter. Another opening, the urethra, provides an exit route for the urine out of the body. The *trigone* is a triangular space at the base of the bladder where the ureters enter the bladder.

An average bladder holds more than 250 ml of urine before producing the desire to urinate.

Contraction of the bladder and *internal sphincter* is an involuntary action, whereas the action of the *external sphincter* is controlled by you. The act of preventing or concluding *voiding* (urination) is learned and voluntary in a healthy body.

Urethra

The *urethra* is a membranous tube that carries urine from the bladder to the exterior of the body. The process of expelling or voiding urine is technically called *micturition*. The external opening of the urethra is the *urethral meatus* or *urinary meatus*. The female urethra is about 1 ½ inches long, and its only function is urination. In the male, it is approximately 8 inches long. It extends from the bladder neck through the prostate and through the penis. The male urethra carries both urine and reproductive organ secretions (see Chapter 22). Thanks to Mother Nature, the urethra can't mix sperm and urine, so it's difficult to pee with an erection. That sure prevents unwanted embarrassment during those tender moments.

Catheter comes from the Greek *catheter*, meaning "a thing let down." A catheter lets down urine from the bladder.

Filtration, reabsorption, and secretion . . . oh, my!

As blood passes through the glomeruli of each kidney, the process of forming urine begins. There are three steps to this process: filtration, reabsorption, and secretion. Glomerular walls are thin to permit water, salt, sugar, and nitrogenous waste such as urea, creatinine, and uric acid to filter out of the blood. Each kidney is surrounded by a cup-like structure that collects the substances filtering out of the blood. This cup-like structure is called *Bowman's capsule*.

If the process of forming urine stopped here, the body would lose a great deal of needed water, sugar, and salt that would be filtered out of the blood with the waste. Each Bowman's capsule is connected to a long twisted tube called a *renal tubule*. As the water, salt, and waste pass through this tubule, the materials that the body needs are able to re-enter the bloodstream through tiny capillaries. By the time the filtrated

material reaches the end of the renal tubule, the materials that the body needs to keep have been re-absorbed.

The waste, along with some water, salt and acids, passes from the renal tubule into the central collecting area of the kidney. Thousands of tubules deposit urine into the *central renal pelvis*, a space that fills most of the medulla of the kidney. Cup-like divisions of the renal pelvis called *calyces* (singular *calyx*) receive the urine, which is (as we mention earlier) made up of 95 percent water, plus 5 percent urea, creatinine, acids, and salts. The renal pelvis narrows into the ureter that carries the urine to the urinary bladder, where it is temporarily stored. When the bladder reaches its capacity, the urge or need to void (urinate) is felt and urine is expelled from the bladder via the urethra. Then, it's off to the bathroom you go!

Micturate comes from the Latin *mictus*, which means "a making of water." From the verb *micturate* comes the noun *micturition*. Be sure to note the spelling: *Micturition* (expelling urine) is often misspelled as *micturation*.

The *p* is silent in *pneumonia*, just as pee is silent in a swimming pool. That's why you probably should not frequent swim-up bars on vacation. You never know what is lurking in the water.

Urinary Root Words

Now it's time to turn on the flow (pun *entirely* intended) of prefixes, suffixes, and root words. In the case of the prefixes and suffixes, you will find that these beginnings and endings of urinary words tend to allude to some sort of condition or state of the urinary system. Table 21-1 gets you started with prefixes and suffixes.

Table 21-1	Starting and Stopping the Flow: Urinary Prefixes and Suffixes
Prefix	**What It Means**
An-	Without
Dys-	Difficult, painful
Poly	Many, much
Trans-	Through or across
Suffix	**What It Means**
-continence	To stop
-emia	A blood condition
-graphy	Process of recording
-iasis	Condition
-itis	Inflammation
-lysis	Loosening, separating
-megaly	Enlargement
-ptosis	Drooping, sagging, prolapse
-tripsy	Surgical crushing
-uria	Urination, urine

Now that you know your urinary prefixes and suffixes coming and going, you can get to the heart of these wee words. Table 21-2 is a list of the most common root words and combining forms in the world of all things urinary.

Table 21-2	To Pee or Not to Pee: Urinary Root Words
Root Word	**What It Means**
Albumin/o	Albumin
Bacteri/o	Bacteria
Cortic/o	Cortex (the renal cortex is the outer section of the kidney)
Crypt/o	Hidden
Cyst/o	Urinary bladder
Dips/o	Thirst
Glomerul/o	Glomerulus (cluster of small vessels)
Hydr/o	Water

Root Word	What It Means
Lith/o	Stone
Meat/o	Meatus
Medull/o	Medulla inner section of the kidney
Nephr/o	Kidney
Noct/i	Night
Olig/o	Scanty
Pyel/o	Renal pelvis
Py/o	Pus
Ren/o	Kidney
Trigon/o	Trigone
Ur/o, urin/o	Urine, urea, urinary tract
Ureter/o	Ureter (you have two)
Urethr/o	Urethra (you have one)

To keep your urethra and ureters straight, remember that ureter has two *es*, and urethra has one *e*. You have two ureters and one urethra.

Common Urinary Conditions

Ah, your urinary system. So few parts, yet so many possible things that can go wrong. Who hasn't enjoyed a few days on the cranberry juice diet thanks to an inconvenient and painful bladder infection? And who could forget the joys of passing a good, old-fashioned kidney stone? Good times — not so much.

When you are dealing with common conditions, remember that inflammation is the arch nemesis of the urinary system. When your urinary parts are inflamed, bacteria has a perfect place to grow amidst a system transporting waste material. This results in infection and a great deal of discomfort. Here are some of the usual suspects:

- ✔ **Cystitis:** Inflammation of the bladder
- ✔ **Ureteritis:** Inflammation of a ureter
- ✔ **Urethritis:** Inflammation of the urethra
- ✔ **Urinary tract infection (UTI):** Infection of one or more organs of the urinary tract

Finding the Culprit: Urinary Diseases and Pathology

Although the typical urinary conditions can cause inconvenience and discomfort, they are sometimes signposts for more serious pathological conditions and diseases. These more serious issues range from diseases that affect kidney function to various varieties of cancer:

- **CRF (chronic renal failure):** When kidney function is not sufficient, leading to dialysis or transplantation

- **Cystocele:** Protrusion or sagging of the bladder

- **End-stage renal disease (ESRD):** Chronic irreversible renal (kidney) failure

- **Epispadias:** Congenital defect in which the urinary meatus is located on the upper surface of penis; usually corrected surgically shortly after birth

- **Essential hypertension:** High blood pressure without apparent cause

- **Glomerulonephritis:** Inflammation of kidney glomeruli caused by any number of things, including connective tissue diseases like *lupus*, endocrine diseases like diabetes, or bacterial infection like untreated *Group A Betahemolytic Streptococcus*

- **Hydronephrosis:** Water or fluid distention in the renal pelvis caused by obstruction of the ureter

- **Hydroureter:** Distention of ureter with urine due to blockage

- **Hypernephroma:** Renal carcinoma in adults

- **Hypospadias:** Congenital defect in which the urinary meatus is located on the under side of the penis; usually corrected surgically as well

- **Incontinence:** Inability to prevent voiding of urine

- **Nephritis:** Inflammation of the kidney

- **Nephroblastoma:** Kidney tumor containing developing cells (*Wilms' tumor*)

- **Nephrolith:** Kidney stone

- **Nephrolithiasis:** Kidney stones or renal calculi

- **Nephroma:** Tumor of the kidney

- **Nephromegaly:** Enlargement of the kidney

- **Nephroptosis:** Drooping or fallen kidney

✔ **Nephrotic syndrome:** Condition due to excessive protein loss in urine

✔ **Nephrosis:** Any disease of the kidney

✔ **Polycystic disease:** Multiple fluid-filled sacs (cysts) in the kidneys

✔ **Pyelitis:** Inflammation of the renal pelvis

✔ **Pyelonephritis:** Inflammation of renal pelvis

✔ **Renal calculi:** Stones in the kidney

✔ **Renal cell carcinoma:** Malignancy of kidney involving the *renal parenchyma* (all its essential parts)

✔ **Renal colic:** Pain due to blockage during passage of a kidney stone

✔ **Renal hypertension:** High blood pressure resulting from kidney disease (secondary hypertension)

✔ **Wilms' tumor:** Malignant kidney tumor, occurs in childhood; also known as adenomyosarcoma

✔ **Transitional cell carcinoma:** Malignancy affecting bladder, ureters, and renal pelvis

✔ **Urinary retention:** Blockage in passage of urine or muscle control problems leading to incomplete voiding with the same result

✔ **Urinary incontinence:** Inability to hold urine in the bladder

Testing, Testing: Urinary Radiology and Diagnostic Tests

Testing the urinary system for diseases and pathological conditions is a bit more involved than peeing in a cup and sending the sample off to the lab. Physicians can prescribe all kinds of tests to root out the problems that affect your plumbing.

First, let's start with some of the tests that do involve the old reliable urine sample. These tests are part of a total *urinalysis* (microscopic analysis of urine), also known as the *UA*, or blood screening process to evaluate adequate functioning of the urinary system:

✔ **Addis count:** Urine test to determine kidney disease; total volume measurement of urine output in 24-hour period is used to evaluate kidney function

Excessive bilirubins can cause *jaundice* in newborns.

✔ **BUN (blood, urea, nitrogen):** Measures amount of urea in the blood; when kidney is diseased or fails, urea accumulates, leading to unconsciousness and death

✔ **CCT (creatinine clearance test):** Measures the ability of the kidney to remove *creatinine,* a white crystallized compound, from the blood

✔ **Phenylketonuria (PKU):** Substance found in urine of newborns indicating congenital problems (routinely performed on newborns)

Physicians might also recommend diagnostic imaging or X-rays to be performed on the urinary system. These imaging procedures are, for the most part, non-invasive with the exception of having to add *contrast media* (often a dye) to the body so that problems show up on the X-ray. Some common diagnostic imaging procedures include the following:

✔ **CAT scan:** Stands for *Computerized Axial Tomography*; a transverse X-ray of kidneys to diagnosis tumors, cysts, abscesses, and hydronephrosis

✔ **Cystogram:** X-ray of bladder

✔ **Cystopyelogram:** X-ray of bladder and renal pelvis

✔ **Cystourethrogram:** X-ray of bladder and urethra

✔ **IVP (intravenous pyelogram):** Injection of contrast media into a vein that travels to the kidneys where it is filtered into the urine; X-rays show the dye filling the kidneys, ureters, bladder, and urethra to diagnose stones, tumors, and cysts

✔ **KUB (kidneys, ureters, bladder):** Demonstrates the size and location of kidneys in relationship to other organs in abdominal and pelvic regions

✔ **Nephrogram:** X-ray of kidney

✔ **Pyelogram:** X-ray of renal pelvis

✔ **Retrograde pyelogram:** Contrast media is injected into the bladder and ureters through a cystoscope; X-rays are taken determine the presence of stones or obstruction

✔ **Ultrasonography (ultrasound):** Kidney size, tumors, hydronephrosis, polycystic kidney, and ureteral/bladder obstructions are some of conditions diagnosed by using sound waves

✔ **Voiding cystogram:** Bladder is filled with contrast media; X-rays are taken of bladder and urethra as urine is expelled

And now for the fun part — endoscopy! Though the following procedures might create some feelings of reservation, just remember that if your physician cannot properly diagnose it, he or she cannot treat it. So, buck up, put on your big girl/big boy pants, and get over your fear of the scope. Some of the most common urinary endoscopic procedures are these:

- **Cystoscope:** Instrument used to visually examine the bladder
- **Cystoscopy:** Visual examination of the bladder
- **Nephroscopy:** Visual examination of the kidney
- **Urethroscope:** Instrument used to visually examine the urethra
- **Urethroscopy:** Visual examination of the urethra
- **Ureteroscope:** Instrument used to visually examine the ureter
- **Ureteroscopy:** Visual examination of the ureter
- **Urinometer:** Instrument used to measure the specific gravity of urine

Paging Dr. Terminology: Urinary Surgeries and Procedures

A plethora of surgeries and procedures are available to help treat disorders and diseases. Like procedures for other body systems, these most often involve excisions, incisions, and repairs. Think of your surgeon as the master plumber of human pipes. These are some typical procedures used in fixing your peeing parts:

- **Cystectomy:** Surgical excision of the bladder
- **Cystoplasty:** Surgical repair of the bladder
- **Cystostomy:** Creation of an artificial opening to the bladder
- **Cystotomy:** Incision into the bladder
- **Fulguration:** Destruction of living tissue with an electric spark, used to remove bladder growth or small tumor
- **Dialysis:** Does the work that a nonfunctioning kidney can't, removes waste material such as urea from the bloodstream
- **ESWL:** Extracorporeal (outside the body) shock wave lithotripsy
- **Hemodialysis:** Artificial kidney machine filters waste from blood
- **Lithotripsy:** Surgical or shock wave disintegration or crushing of kidney stones
- **Nephrectomy:** Surgical excision of a kidney

- **Nephrolysis:** Separation of the kidneys from other body structures

- **Nephrolithotomy:** Surgical removal of a kidney stone through incision into the kidney

- **Nephropexy:** Surgical fixation of a kidney

- **Peritoneal dialysis:** Waste is removed from the blood via fluid exchange through the peritoneal cavity

- **Pyelolithotomy:** Incision into the renal pelvis to remove stones

- **Pyeloplasty:** Surgical repair of the renal pelvis

- **Renal biopsy:** Biopsy of a kidney performed at time of surgery or through the skin (subcutaneous or closed) in which a needle is inserted with ultrasound guidance; tissue is obtained and later used to diagnose diseases from cancer to diabetes damage

- **Renal transplant:** Surgical implantation of a kidney to replace a nonfunctioning kidney; because each kidney performs the same function, the body can survive with only one kidney

- **Ureterectomy:** Surgical excision a ureter

- **Ureterostomy:** Creating an artificial opening into a ureter; usually used to create an opening from the ureter to the skin so urine can be collected in a bag

- **Ureterotomy:** Incision into a ureter

- **Urethropexy:** Surgical fixation of the urethra

- **Urethrovesical suspension:** Surgical suspension of the bladder and urethra

Terminology RX: Urinary Pharmacology

The medications used most often in the treatment of urinary conditions and diseases are used for lots of other bodily issues. You will no doubt recognize these drug families, as they are crossover drugs.

Traditional antibiotics are typically used to treat urinary tract infections. These drugs are most effective against gram-negative E. coli organisms, the common culprits in UTIs (urinary tract infections). *Gram-negative* is a negative response to a *Gram's stain*, a staining method to detect microorganisms. Though drinking a lot of cranberry juice is helpful when you have an uncomfortable UTI, it is not a panacea. Rely on prescription antibiotics to really wipe out the infection and get your pee flowing again. Another type of drug common in treating urinary tract infections is the family of *sulfonamides*.

Diuretics, often taken for hypertension, make the kidneys work overtime. A potassium (K) supplement is often given to maintain therapeutic potassium levels in the blood. A diuretic increases the excretion of urine, putting the entire urinary system into overdrive, which is not good for the kidneys or for sodium and potassium levels. This is why great caution is exercised when prescribing these drugs, and all drugs in this family are by prescription only. There are some common, everyday items that have diuretic effects, such as the caffeine in your coffee or soda.

Urinary odds and ends: Additional vocabulary

We couldn't leave this chapter without including some useful terms that don't necessarily fit into our usual categories. Drumroll, please . . . we give you a urinary grab bag (not to be confused with the urinary catheter bag). Commit these potpourri urinary words to memory, and you'll be the star of the doctor's office:

- **Anuria:** Absence of urine

- **Azotemia:** Excessive urea and nitrogen in the blood

- **Azoturia:** Excessive urea and nitrogen in urine

- **Catheter:** A flexible tube-like device for withdrawing or instilling fluid

- **Diuresis:** Increased excretion of urine

- **Diuretic:** An agent or medication used to increase the amount of urine production (water pill)

- **Dysuria:** Difficulty or painful urination

- **Enuresis:** Bedwetting

- **Glycosuria:** Sugar or glucose in urine

- **Hematuria:** Blood in urine

- **Nephrologist:** Physician who specializes in treating kidney disease

- **Nephrology:** The study of the kidney, its anatomy and functions

- **Nocturia:** Night urination

- **Oliguria:** Scanty urination

- **Polyuria:** Excessive urination

- **Pyuria:** Pus in urine

- **Urinary:** Pertaining to urine

- **Urologist:** Physician who specializes in treating diseases of the male and female urinary system and male reproductive system

- **Urology:** The study of the male and female urinary system and male reproductive system

- **Urinary catheterization:** Passage of a catheter through the urethra into the bladder to withdraw urine

Chapter 22

Check the Plumbing: Male Reproductive System

*T*hey say it takes two to tango. You can't create life without input from both the male and the female reproductive organs. Both are equally important to the process of babymaking, which is why they each get their own chapter in this book. Normally, we would say, "Ladies first," but in this case, let's start our reproductive discussion with the guys, who donate the "little soldiers" responsible for egg fertilization.

How the Male Reproductive System Works

The reproductive system in the male has two main functions, to produce *spermatozoa* (singular: *spermatozoon*), the male reproductive cells, and to secrete *testosterone*, the male hormone. The male reproductive organs, or gonads, are the *testes*. They are supported by accessory organs, ducts, and glands. The ducts include the *epididymides* (singular: *epididymis*) *vas deferens*, *ejaculatory ducts*, and the *urethra*. Glands include *seminal vesicles*, *prostate*, and *bulbourethral glands* (or *Cowper's glands*). The supporting structures include the *penis*, *scrotum*, and *spermatic cords*.

The spermatozoon is called *sperm* for short. Each sperm is a microscopic cell, measuring less than 1/100,000th the size of the female *ovum*. Its structure is uncomplicated, composed of a head region that contains the hereditary material, or *chromosomes*, and a tail. This tail region, called the *flagellum*, is a hair-like structure that makes the sperm *motile* (able to move by itself), resembling a tadpole.

The sperm cell contains little food and cytoplasm, because a sperm only needs to live long enough to travel from its point of release in the male to where the ovum (egg cell) lies in the female in the *fallopian tube*. Only one spermatozoon can penetrate a single egg and achieve fertilization. Imagine, of the approximately 300–500 *million* spermatozoa that can be released in a single ejaculation, only one can complete the fertilization process.

The male reproductive system produces 100 million sperm per day (that's a rate of 1,000 for every heartbeat), from puberty until death! The organs of the male reproductive system are designed to produce and release billions of spermatozoa throughout the male's lifetime.

In addition, the male reproductive system secretes the male hormone (or *androgen*) testosterone. Testosterone is necessary for the proper development of the male gonads from the fetal stage through adulthood, the testes or testicles (singular: *testis*) and accessory organs of the testes, the prostate gland, and seminal vesicles. Testosterone is also responsible for the production of secondary body characteristics of the male, such as a facial hair and voice deepening. The prostate gland and seminal vesicles secrete fluid to ensure the sperm cells' lubrication and *viability* (the ability to live).

Figure 22-1 takes a look at this system's anatomy, and the organs and parts that make up the system.

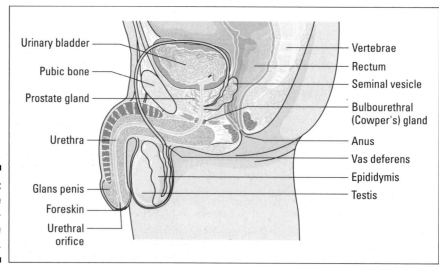

Figure 22-1:
The male reproductive anatomy.

From LifeARTS®, Super Anatomy 1, ©2002, Lippincott Williams & Wilkins

Testes

The male *gonads* consist of two *testes* or *testicles*, which are egg-shaped glands that develop in the kidney region before descending into the scrotum before birth.

The interior of a testis is composed of a large mass of narrow coiled tubules called the *seminiferous tubules*. These contain cells that manufacture spermatozoa. These tubules are the *parenchymal tissue* of the testis, meaning they perform the essential work of the organ. Other cells in the testis, called *interstitial cells* (or *Leydig cells*), manufacture the male hormone testosterone. These tubules come together and enter the head of the *epididymis*.

The *scrotum* is a sac enclosing the testes on the outside of the body. The scrotum lies between the thighs in order to expose the testes to a lower temperature than if they were enclosed within the body. This lower temperature is necessary for the adequate maturing and development of sperm.

Between the anus and the scrotum, at the floor of the pelvic cavity in the male is the *perineum*, which is similar to the perineal region in the female.

Ducts

Once formed, sperm cells move through the seminiferous tubules and are collected in ducts that lead to a large tube at the upper part of each testis, the *epididymis*. The spermatozoa become motile and move into the epididymis, where they are stored.

The epididymis runs the length of each testicle, is about 20 feet long when uncoiled, and is the passageway for sperm from the testis to the body surface. It stores sperm before ejaculation and secretes a portion of the *seminal fluid* (semen).

The vas deferens are a pair of tubes approximately 0.3 cm in diameter and 2 feet long. The tubes, a continuation of the epididymis, carry the sperm up into the pelvic region and around the urinary bladder, where they connect with the seminal vesicle duct to form the ejaculatory duct. It is the vas deferens that are cut or tied off when a male sterilization procedure, called a *vasectomy*, is performed.

Ejaculatory ducts are formed by the joining of vas deferens with the ducts of the *seminal vesicles*, which are located at the base of the bladder and open into the vas deferens as it joins the urethra. These vesicles secrete a thick yellow substance, seminal fluid, that nourishes the sperm cells and forms much of the volume of the ejaculated semen or seminal fluid.

Urethra

Semen is a combination of fluid and spermatozoa, ejected from the body through the *urethra*. In the male, the *genital orifice* (opening) combines with the urinary urethral opening. The male urethra is part of the urinary system as well as the reproductive system because it aids in the output of both urine and semen.

Cowper's glands, or bulbourethral glands, are just below the prostate gland and also secrete fluid into the urethra. The urethra passes through the penis to exit the body.

Prostate

At the region where the vas deferens enters the urethra, and almost encircling the upper end of the urethra, is the *prostate gland*. This gland secretes a thick alkaline fluid which, as part of the seminal fluid, aids in the motility of the sperm. This gland is also supplied with muscular tissue that aids in the expulsion of sperm during ejaculation. The alkaline also protects the sperm from acid present in the male urethra and the vagina of the female.

Prostate comes from the Greek *pro* meaning "before." *Statis* means "standing"; by anatomy, is the gland standing slightly before and below the bladder.

Penis

The penis is composed of three rounded masses of erectile tissue and at its tip expands to form a soft, sensitive region called the *glans penis*. The glans penis is covered with a retractable double fold of skin called the *prepuce* (foreskin). The penis contains the urethra that carries both seminal fluid and urine. It is the organ by means of which sperm is ejected into the female vagina.

Male Reproductive Root Words

To really stretch a metaphor, as the human race needs both male and female reproductive systems in order to survive by creating new life, the medical terms associated with the male reproductive system need both prefixes and suffixes to create new words.

Table 22-1 lists one prefix and a few suffixes to know when it comes to male reproductive terminology.

Table 22-1	Making Word Babies: Male Reproductive Prefixes and Suffixes
Prefixes or Suffix	**What It Means**
-ism	State of
-ectomy	Surgical removal of
-pexy	Surgical fixation
-itis	Inflammation
-orrhea	Excessive discharge
-plasty	Surgical repair of
Trans-	Through, across, beyond

And now for the glue that holds these medical terms together. Take a look at the root words and combining forms that pertain to this system, shown in Table 22-2.

Table 22-2	Life Force: Male Reproductive System Root Words
Root Word	**What It Means**
Andr/o	Male
Balan/o	Glans penis
Cry/o	Cold
Epididym/o	Epididymis
Orch/o, orchi/o, orchid/o	Testis, testicle
Prostat/o	Prostate gland
Sperm/o	Spermatozoon
Spermat/o	Spermatozoa
Test/o	Testis, testicle
Vas/o	Vessel or duct
Vesicul/o	Seminal vesicles

Common Male Reproductive Conditions

The makeup of the male reproductive system, with all its tubes and ducts, can be complicated and subject to several types of conditions. Here are some of the pathological conditions associated with the male reproductive system:

- **Adenocarcinoma:** Malignant tumor of the prostate; second most common cause of cancer deaths in men over 50; radical (complete) prostatectomy along with radiation and chemotherapy is the most common treatment

- **Andropathy:** Diseases of the male

- **Anorchism:** The state of absence of a testicle, one or both

- **Aspermia:** Condition of absence of sperm

- **Balanocele:** Protrusion of glans penis (through rupture of prepuce)

- **Balanitis:** Inflammation of glans penis

- **Balanorrhea:** Excessive discharge from the glans penis, often the first symptom of a sexually transmitted disease

- **BPH (benign prostatic hypertrophy/hyperplasia):** Enlargement or excessive development of prostate gland in males over 60 years of age, can cause a urinary obstruction with inability to empty the bladder completely or all at once; surgical treatment is *prostatectomy*

- **Cryptorchidism:** Undescended testicle (*crypt* meaning "hidden"); two months before birth, testicles should descend into scrotal sac

- **Epididymitis:** Inflammation of the epididymis

- **Epispadias:** Congenital (present at birth) opening of the male urethra on the upper surface of penis

- **Erectile dysfunction:** Inability of male to attain or maintain an erection to perform sexual intercourse

- **Hydrocele:** Hernia or sac of fluid in the testis or in the tube leading from the testis, can occur in infancy and usually resolves during the first year of life

- **Hypospadias:** Congenital opening of the male urethra on the undersurface of the penis (present at birth)

- **Impotence:** Lack of power to obtain erection or to copulate

- **Oligospermia:** Condition of scanty sperm (in seminal fluid)

- **Orchitis/orchiditis:** Inflammation of testes or a testis

- **Phimosis:** Narrowing of the opening of the foreskin over the glans penis that does not allow the foreskin to retract, obstructing urination and causing secretions to accumulate under the prepuce, leading to infection

- **Priapism:** Prolonged abnormal erection of penis with pain and tenderness

- **Prostatitis:** Inflammation of the prostate gland

- **Prostatocystitis:** Inflammation of prostate gland and bladder

- **Prostatolith:** Stone in the prostate

- **Prostatorrhea:** Excessive discharge from the prostate

- **Testicular torsion:** Twisting of spermatic cord causing decreased blood flow to testicle; occurs most often during puberty; considered a surgical emergency

- **Testicular carcinoma:** Malignant tumor of the testis, classified according to type of tissue involved; examples: *seminoma, embryonal carcinoma,* and *teratocarcinoma* (a malignant *teratoma*); commonly treated with surgery: orchidectomy, radiation, and chemotherapy

- **Varicocele:** Large, herniated, swollen veins near the testis, associated with *oligospermia* (lower than normal amount of sperm) and infertility

Finding the Culprit: Male Reproductive Diseases and Pathology

Unfortunately, some of the most common diseases of the male reproductive system are the kind that make headlines, and not in a good way. Sexually transmitted diseases are very serious, highly contagious, and can affect everything from your ability to conceive to your relationships with future sexual partners.

Also known as *venereal diseases*, the following conditions occur in both male and female and are among the most communicable diseases in the world, transmitted by unprotected sexual intercourse, via body fluids. Here are the usual suspects:

- **AIDS (acquired immunodeficiency syndrome)** is a sexually transmitted disease by exchange of body fluids during a sexual act or with use of contaminated needles and contaminated blood transfusion, affecting the body's immune system. It is caused by HIV (Human Immunodeficiency Virus).

- **Chlamydia,** the bacterium Chlamydia trachomatis, is the causative agent; includes diseases of the eye and genital tract. It causes discharge from the penis in males and genital itching, and vaginal discharge in females. It can cause infertility in women if it spreads to the ovaries and uterus and causes pelvic scarring secondary to the infection.

✔ **Genital herpes** is infection of the skin and mucous membranes of the genitals, caused by Herpesvirus hominis type 2. Symptoms include reddening of the skin with small fluid-filled blisters and ulcers. Remission and relapse periods occur, and no drug is known to be effective as a cure.

✔ **Gonorrhea** is a contagious inflammation of the genital tract mucous membranes due to infection with a bacteria known as Gonococcus. Other areas of the body such as the eye, mouth, rectum, and joints may be affected. Symptoms include *dysuria* (painful urination) and discharge from the urethra. Many women can carry this disease without symptoms, but others have pain, vaginal and urethral discharge. Penicillin is the method of treatment. Ongoing data from the CDC demonstrate that gonorrheal infections have become resistant to *fluoroquinolone* antibiotics such as *ciprofloxacin* and *ofloxacin*. As a consequence, as of 2007 this class of antibiotics is no longer recommended for the treatment of gonorrhea in the United States. The most commonly recommended treatment is an injection of a *cephalosporin* class of antibiotics called *ceftriaxone*.

✔ **Human immunodeficiency virus (HIV)** is the retrovirus causing AIDS. HIV infects T-cell helpers of the immune system, allowing for opportunistic infections like *candidiasis, P. carinii, pneumonia, tuberculosis,* and *Kaposi's sarcoma*.

✔ **Human papilloma virus (HPV)** is a sexually transmitted disease causing benign or cancerous growths in male and female genitals (venereal warts). *Venereal warts* are also known as *condyloma acuminatum* (plural: *condylomata acuminata*).

✔ **Syphilis** is a chronic infectious disease affecting any organ of the body and is caused by a spiral-shaped bacteria. A *chancre*, or hard ulcer, usually appears a few weeks after infection, most often on external genitals but may also be on the lip, tongue, or anus with enlargement of lymph nodes. Infection can spread to internal organs, and later stages include damage to brain, spinal cord, and heart. Syphilis can be *congenital* (existing at birth) to a newborn if transmitted from the mother during pregnancy via the placenta. Penicillin is the method of treatment.

✔ **Trichomoniasis** means infection of the urinary tract of either sex and is caused by the one-cell organism Trichomonas. Males may have no symptoms or could develop *urethritis* (inflammation of the urethra), or prostate enlargement. Females develop itching, dysuria, and vaginal discharge.

Venereal is derived from Venus, the goddess of love. It was thought in ancient times to be one of the misfortunes of love.

Testing, Testing: Male Reproductive Radiology and Diagnostic Tests

It's time to test those testes! Okay, bad pun, but you get the drift. Though there aren't tons of laboratory tests and diagnostic procedures used for this system, they remain important methods for helping men of all ages find peace when it comes to issues of concern related to sexual health.

One very common test is *semen analysis*. This test is performed as part of fertility studies and also to establishment fertility status. Sometimes the test is performed to determine sperm viability for couples having difficulty conceiving. It can also be performed following a vasectomy to assure that the procedure was successful. In this case, semen is collected in a sterile container and analyzed microscopically; sperm cells are counted and examined for motility and shape. Analysis is also done at six weeks following vasectomy and again at three months, to establish aspermia.

Another common test for men is the *GC/Chlamydia test*, performed by inserting a small cotton swab into the opening of the urethra to obtain a sample, which is then tested for gonorrhea and Chlamydia.

A general *viral culture* tests for herpes and HIV, and is performed simply by swabbing an open sore.

In *VDRL*, also known as the *Venereal Disease Research Laboratory test*, the blood is tested to diagnose syphilis. Because the syphilis antigen stays in the blood for a lifetime, it can have far-reaching effects.

The *PSA (prostate specific antigen test)* is recommended to be done yearly on males over 50. This is a prescreening mechanism for precancerous conditions of the prostate gland. Any rise or elevation of PSA level is followed up by other investigations.

Prostate carcinoma is both serious and scary. Any time a disease, particularly cancer, is associated with a reproductive system, it can cause more than just physical symptoms. It can be emotionally and mentally devastating, because we associate our sexual identities with our sexual systems. Much as a woman feels devastated by breast cancer, a man can feel equally devastated by a cancer affecting his sexual health. Prostate cancer is one of the most common cancers associated with the male reproductive system.

Here are some typical prostate carcinoma investigations:

- ✔ **Digital rectal examination (DRE)** of prostate
- ✔ **Prostate specific antigen (PSA)** blood test
- ✔ **Transrectal ultrasound/ultrasound examination** of prostate through the rectum using sound waves

Paging Dr. Terminology: Male Reproductive Surgeries and Procedures

You've found the problem, now it's time to call the plumber, or, in this case, the urologist. Take a look at some of the procedural terms you'll need to know about all things male:

- ✔ **Balanoplasty:** Surgical repair of the glans penis
- ✔ **Circumcision:** Surgery to remove the foreskin (prepuce) from the penis; usually performed on newborn male but can be performed in adult males for *phimosis* (narrowing of the opening of the foreskin over the glans penis obstructing urination and causing secretions to accumulate under the foreskin, leading to infection)
- ✔ **Hydrocelectomy:** Surgical removal of a hydrocele
- ✔ **Orchidectomy:** Surgical removal of one or both testes (if both, called *castration*)
- ✔ **Orchidopexy:** Surgical fixation or "stitching in place" of a testicle
- ✔ **Orchioplasty:** Surgical repair of testis
- ✔ **Penile implant:** Surgical implanting of a penile prosthesis to correct erectile dysfunction (*prosthesis* means "artificial body part")
- ✔ **Prostatectomy:** Excision of prostate gland
- ✔ **TUMT (transurethral microwave thermotherapy):** A *prostatron* is used to deliver microwaves heating the area for one hour, to eliminate excessive tissue present in BPH; no anesthetic required
- ✔ **TURP (transurethral resection of prostate):** *Resection* (removal of part or all of the gland) through the urethra; cutting back or removal of the prostate if enlargement of the prostate may interfere with urination
- ✔ **Vasectomy:** Excision of a portion of the vas deferens to perform male sterilization; vas deferens on each side is cut, a portion removed, and the free ends are tied off or clipped, done through an incision in the

scrotum; sterilizes the male in a way that sperm is not released with the seminal fluid; does not interfere with nerves or blood supply to the testis or penis; hormone secretions, sex drive, and potency not affected

Terminology RX: Male Reproductive Pharmacology

Believe it or not, there is more to male reproductive pharmacology that that infamous pill to aid in *erectile dysfunction*. However, that pill certainly is nice, and you will wow all of your friends by knowing its official generic name, which is *sildenafil citrate*. *Vasodilators* like this keep things cooking in the bedroom for those who are experiencing difficulty.

Everything you ever wanted to know about male reproductive vocabulary but were afraid to ask

For the final push of this chapter, we spill all some additional vocabulary words you may need to know to speak definitively about the male reproductive system, while refreshing your memory on a few others. Here is the crazy mix of words that help you understand this system:

✔ **Aspermia:** Absence of sperm

✔ **Artificial insemination:** Introduction of semen in to the vagina by artificial means

✔ **Coitus/copulation:** Sexual intercourse between male and female

✔ **Condom:** Protective covering for the penis, worn during coitus

✔ **Ejaculation:** Male orgasm, ejection of seminal fluid from the male urethra

✔ **Genitalia:** Reproductive organs

✔ **Gonads:** Male and female sex glands; in the male, testes; in the female, ovaries

✔ **Heterosexual:** A person who is attracted to the opposite sex

✔ **Homosexual:** A person who is attracted to the same sex

✔ **Impotence:** Inability to achieve or maintain an erection or to copulate

✔ **Oligospermia:** Scanty amount of sperm in seminal fluid

✔ **Orgasm:** Climax of sexual intercourse

✔ **Penis:** The male organ of copulation or sexual intercourse and the means by which sperm travels from the male to the female; considered an accessory organ of the reproductive system

✔ **Polyorchism:** Presence of more than two testes

✔ **Puberty:** Period when secondary sex characteristics develop and ability to reproduce sexually begins

✔ **Sterilization:** The process that renders person unable to produce offspring

The usual routine for any inflammations is antibiotics, and it's no different for the male reproductive system.

Finally, on a more serious note, *amebicides*, *antifungal agents*, as well as good old penicillin are used to treat the STD family of bacteria. Amebicides treat amebal infections, almost always of the intestines; fungicides treat fungi, most commonly *tinea cruris*, or jock itch; penicillin is still the treatment for syphilis.

Chapter 23

A Life Force: The Female Reproductive System

*I*f you thought the male reproductive system was complicated, you ain't seen nothin' yet, baby! Not only is the female system the other half of the reproductive puzzle that helps create a human life, it is also the vessel that helps sustain that little life in the nine months prior to birth. It's the docking station where sperm and egg meet and the storage facility for the end product. That's a lot of pressure to put on one system — create life, sustain new life, and nurture new life. Oh yeah, not to mention the business of squeezing something the size of a cantaloupe out of something the size of a mango.

How the Female Reproductive System Works

The female reproductive system produces the female reproductive cell, or sex cell, secretes the hormones estrogen and progesterone, and provides the conditions to establish a pregnancy, together with providing a safe place for the pregnancy to develop and grow.

The *gonads* (the *ovaries* in the female), together with the internal accessory organs consisting of the *fallopian (uterine) tubes*, *uterus*, *vagina*, *external genitalia*, and *breasts (mammary glands)* make up the reproductive system in the female. Reproduction is achieved by the union of the female reproductive cell, an *ovum*, and the male reproductive cell, a *spermatozoon* (or *sperm* for short), resulting in *fertilization*.

Gynecology is the study of the organs, hormones, and diseases of the female reproductive system. *Obstetrics* is the specialty dealing with care of the female during pregnancy and delivery of the newborn, including the 6–8-week period following delivery.

The female and male sex cells (ovum and sperm), differ from normal body cells. Each sex cell, also called a *gamete*, is a specialized cell, containing half the number of chromosomes (23) of a normal body cell (46). As the ovum and sperm cells unite, the resulting cell produced, called the *zygote*, contains half the genetic material from the female sex cell and half from the male sex cell. This combination provides a full normal complement of hereditary material.

Take a closer look now at the working parts of the female system in Figure 23-1.

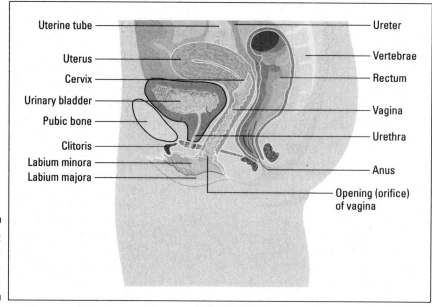

Figure 23-1:
The female reproductive system.

From LifeARTS®, Super Anatomy 1, ©2002, Lippincott Williams & Wilkins

Ovaries

The *ovaries* are two almond-shaped glands, located on either side of the uterus in the pelvic cavity. They are held in place and connected to the uterus by the *broad* and *ovarian ligaments*. These organs have two functions: First, they release a mature ovum each month in a process known as ovulation. They also produce and secrete the sex hormones, estrogen and progesterone. *Estrogen* secretion begins development of female secondary sex characteristics, as well as manages the cyclic or menstrual changes in the uterus, preparing for a fertilized ovum. *Progesterone* is produced in the *corpus luteum* of the ovary and in the placenta in order to support and nurture a fertilized ovum.

Each ovary contains thousands of sacs called graafian follicles. Each of these follicles contains an ovum. As an ovum matures, the graafian follicle ruptures to the surface and the ovum leaves the ovary. The ruptured follicle fills with blood and yellow material and becomes a *corpus luteum*. Near each ovary is a duct-like tube called the fallopian tube. The fallopian tubes and ovaries are called the *adnexa*, or accessory structures of the uterus.

The graafian follicle is named after Reinier de Graaf, a Dutch anatomist who discovered the graafin sac in 1672.

Figure 23-2 shows the menstrual cycle.

Fallopian tubes

The *fallopian tubes* lead from each ovary to the uterus.

The ovum, after its release, is caught up by *fimbriae*, the finger-like projections at the end of the fallopian tube. The tube is lined with small hairs that, through their motion, sweep the ovum in a process that takes approximately five days to allow that ovum to pass through the fallopian tube. Fertilization takes place within the fallopian tube if spermatozoa are present. If intercourse has taken place near the time of ovulation, and no contraception is used, sperm cells will be in the fallopian tube when the ovum passes through. If intercourse has not taken place, and the ovum is not fertilized, it will disintegrate.

Fallopian tubes are named after Italian anatomist Gabriele Falloppio (1523–1562). He was also responsible for naming the vagina and placenta. We sure wouldn't want to be his kid. Heaven only knows what he might name you.

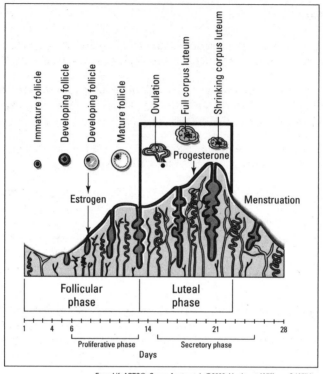

Figure 23-2:
The
menstrual
cycle.

Uterus

When fertilization occurs anytime between puberty and menopause, the fertilized ovum will grow and develop in the *uterus*. Hormones (estrogen and progesterone) are secreted from the ovary, and the HCG hormone is secreted from the placenta, the blood-vessel-filled organ that grows in the wall of the uterus during a pregnancy.

The *uterus* is a muscular organ located between the bladder and the rectum. The uterus is pear-shaped, with muscular walls and a mucous membrane lining with a rich supply of blood vessels. The upper rounded portion of the uterus is called the *fundus*, and the large central portion is called the *corpus* or *body*. It is within the body and fundus of the uterus that a pregnancy grows. The *epithelial mucosa* of the uterus is more commonly called the *endometrium*. The muscular layer is the *myometrium* in the middle, and the outer membranous tissue layer is the *perimetrium*. The narrow lower portion of the uterus is called the *cervix*, meaning "neck." The cervix has an opening at its lower end, leading to the vagina (birth canal), which opens to the outside of the body.

Vagina

The *vagina* is a muscular tube approximately 6 inches long and lined with mucous membrane. The entrance to the vagina is called the *introitus*.

The *clitoris* is situated in front of the vaginal opening and the *urethral meatus*. The clitoris is similar in structure to the penis in the male, being an organ made up of sensitive, erectile tissue.

Bartholin's glands are two small glands on each side of the vaginal opening. They produce a mucous secretion that lubricates the vagina.

Bartholin's gland is named after Caspar Thomeson Bartholin, a Danish anatomist (1655–1738).

The region between the vaginal opening and the anus is called the *perineum*. This may be torn during the process of childbirth in a vaginal delivery. To avoid a perineal tear, the perineum may be cut prior to delivery. This incision is called an *episiotomy*.

The external genitalia (organs of reproduction) of the female are together called the *vulva*. The *labia majora* are the outer lips of the vagina, and the *labia minora* are the smaller inner lips. The *hymen* is a mucous membrane partially covering the entrance to the vagina. The clitoris and Bartholin's glands are also part of the vulva.

Time to accessorize!

The *breasts* are considered accessory organs of the reproduction system. They are *mammary*, or milk-producing glands, composed of fatty tissue, *lactiferous* or *milk-carrying ducts*, and sinus cavities, which carry milk to the opening or nipple. The breast nipple is called the *mammary papilla*, and the dark pigmented area around the nipple is the *areola*.

During a pregnancy, hormones from the ovaries and placenta stimulate gland tissue in the breasts to their full development. After *parturition* (giving birth), hormones from the pituitary gland stimulate milk production in a process known as *lactation*.

There are two hormones involved in milk production: *oxytocin* and *prolactin*. These hormones also work to assist during labor, delivery, and the recovery of the mother. Oxytocin stimuates the uterus to contract, inducing parturition. Following delivery, oxytocin helps contract the uterus back to its normal size. It also reacts on the breasts to stimulate the release of milk. Prolactin stimulates breast development and the formation of milk in the postpartum period. The act of sucking promotes prolactin production, which in turn, promotes further milk production.

Female Reproductive Root Words

So, for lack of a better metaphor, prefixes and suffixes combined with root words are kind of like ova and sperm. Separately, they don't make much sense. But together, they produce a whole new being. In this case, of course, it's a word and not a baby. But they *are* cute, aren't they?

Table 23-1 lists some pertinent prefixes and suffixes.

Table 23-1	Half of the Puzzle: Female Reproductive Prefixes and Suffixes
Prefix	*What It Means*
Dys-	Painful, difficult
Hydro-	Water
Intra-	Within
Nulli-	None
Peri-	Around
Primi-	First
Secundi-	Second
Suffix	*What It Means*
-cyesis	Pregnancy
-ectomy	Surgical removal of
-itis	Inflammation
-optosis	Sagging
-orrhaphy	Suture
-orrhea	Discharge, flow
-oscopy	Visual examination
-plasty	Surgical repair
-rrhagia	Burst forth, excessive flow
-salpinx	Fallopian tube
-tocia	Labor

By adding in the root words and combining forms, you start to create your own little word babies. If you've ever spent any time at the OB-GYN's office, even as a patient, you will probably recognize many of the female-related roots shown in Table 23-2.

Table 23-2	Life-Giving Roots of the Female Reproductive System
Root Word	*What It Means*
Amni/o	Amniocentesis
Cephal/o	Head
Cervic/o	Cervix/neck
Chori/o	Relationship to a membrane
Colp/o	Vagina
Cyes/o, cyes/i	Pregnancy
Episi/o	Vulva
Embry/o	Embryo
Fet/o	Fetus
Fimbri/o	Fimbria
Galact/o	Milk
Gravida	Pregnancy
Gynec/o	Woman, female
Hyster/o	Uterus
Lact/o	Milk
Mamm/o, mast/o	Breast
Men/o	Menstruation
Metr/o, metr/io	Uterus
Mult/i	Many
My/o	Muscle
Nat/o	Birth
Null/i	None
Omphal/o	Umbilicus, navel
Oophor/o	Ovary
Ov/o	Egg, ovum
Pelv/i, pelv/o	Pelvis
Perine/o	Perineum
Prim/i	First
Pseud/o	False
Puerper/o	Childbirth
Salping/o	Fallopian tube

Table 23-2 *(continued)*	
Root Word	*What It Means*
Vagin/o	Vagina
Vulv/o	Vulva
Umbilic/o	Umbilicus, navel
Uter/o	Uterus

It's All Related: More Female Reproductive Anatomical Terms

There are so many medical terms associated with the female reproductive system that it's just not possible, especially in a book this size, to classify each and every one of them. In the following section we provide a diverse array of both anatomical and clinical words that will keep you in the know regarding this system.

- **Adnexa:** Accessory parts of an organ
- **Anteversion:** Abnormal tipping forward of the uterus
- **Coitus/copulation:** Sexual intercourse
- **Estrogen:** Hormone produced by the ovaries responsible for female sex characteristics and building of uterine lining during the menstrual cycle
- **Gynopathic:** Pertaining to diseases of women
- **Hydrosalpinx:** Water in the fallopian tube
- **Leukorrhea:** White vaginal discharge, can sometimes contain white blood cells
- **Mastoptosis:** Sagging breasts
- **Myometrium:** Muscular layer lining the uterus
- **Oligomenorrhea:** Scanty menstrual flow
- **Orifice:** Opening
- **Progesterone:** Hormone produced by the corpus luteum in the ovary and by the placenta during pregnancy
- **Puberty:** Beginning of the fertile period when gametes are produced and secondary sex characteristics become evident
- **Retroversion:** Abnormal tipping backward of the uterus
- **Salpingitis:** Inflammation of fallopian tube

Full circle: The mysteries of the 28-day menstrual cycle revealed

What actually happens on a monthly basis once menstruation begins?

At puberty the beginning of menstruation is called *menarche*, which can begin as early as age nine or as late as 15–16. Every menstrual cycle is divided into approximately 28 days (give or take, depending on your body's makeup) that can be grouped into four time periods:

✔ **Days 1–5, menstrual period:** Bloody fluid containing disintegrated *endometrial* cells and blood cells is discharged through the vagina.

✔ **Days 6–13, postmenstrual period:** When the menstrual period has ended, the lining of the uterus begins to repair itself as the hormone *estrogen* is released by the maturing *graafian follicle (developing egg sac).*

✔ **Days 13–14, ovulation:** The graafian follicle ruptures, and the ovum leaves the ovary and is pulled into the fallopian tube.

✔ **Days 15–28, premenstrual period:** The empty graafian follicle fills with a yellow material and becomes known as a *corpus luteum.* The corpus luteum acts like an endocrine organ and secretes two hormones, estrogen and progesterone, into the bloodstream. The hormones stimulate buildup of the lining of the uterus in preparation for a fertilized ovum. If fertilization does not occur, the corpus luteum stops hormone production and regresses. The fall in hormonal levels leads to the breakdown of the *uterine endometrium,* and a new menstrual cycle begins, bringing the cycle back to day 1.

If fertilization does occur in the fallopian tube, the fertilized ovum moves into the uterus and implants in the *endometrium.* The corpus luteum continues to produce progesterone and estrogen, which supports the vascular and muscular development of the uterus lining. The *placenta,* the organ of communication between the mother and the embryo, now forms in the uterine wall. The placenta produces its own hormone as it develops in the uterus, called *human chorionic gonadotropin (HCG).* HCG is the hormone tested for in the urine of women who suspect a pregnancy. When you pee on a pregnancy test stick, this is the hormone that makes that little plus sign appear. If you see it, pour yourself a champagne glass full of milk and celebrate — you're pregnant!

Some medical terms are specific to the *obstetrical* nature of this system. If you'll be spending any time in an OB's office, whether as an employee or patient, these are some handy terms to know:

✔ **Antepartum:** Before birth, in relation to the mother

✔ **Congenital anomaly:** An abnormality or defect present at birth

✔ **Ectopic:** Occurring away from a normal position

✔ **Ectopic pregnancy:** Pregnancy occurring in the fallopian tube

✔ **Embryo:** The product of conception up to the eight-week period of gestation

✔ **Fetus:** The embryo from second month of pregnancy to delivery

✔ **Pseudocyesis:** False pregnancy

✔ **Hyperemesis gravidarum:** Excessive vomiting during pregnancy

✔ **Gravida:** A pregnant female

✔ **Galactorrhea:** Discharge of milk from the breast

✔ **Intrapartum:** During labor and delivery, in relation to the mother

✔ **Lochia:** The vaginal discharge after childbirth

✔ **Meconium:** First stool of the newborn

✔ **Multigravida:** Female who has been pregnant two or more times

✔ **Multipara:** Female who has given birth to viable offspring two or more times

✔ **Neonate:** A newborn infant from birth to four weeks of age

✔ **Neonatologist:** A physician specializing in neonatology

✔ **Neonatology:** The study, diagnosis, and treatment of disorders of the newborn infant up to one month of age

✔ **Nulligravida:** Female who has never been pregnant

✔ **Nullipara:** A woman who has never given birth

✔ **Parturition:** The act of giving birth

✔ **Postnatal:** Period after birth, referring to the newborn

✔ **Postpartum:** After delivery, in relation to the mother

✔ **Prenatal:** Period before birth, referring to the fetus

✔ **Primipara:** A woman who has given birth to viable offspring for the first time

✔ **Primigravida:** Female who is pregnant for the first time

✔ **Puerpera:** A woman who has just given birth

✔ **Puerperium:** Period after delivery until reproductive organs return to normal, about six to eight weeks

✔ **Quickening:** Female's first awareness of movement of fetus within the uterus, usually felt at approximately 18 weeks' gestation

✔ **Secundigravida:** Female pregnant for the second time

✔ **Secundipara:** Female who has given birth to viable offspring for the second time

Common Female Reproductive Conditions

There's more to the female reproductive system than making babies. With all that equipment, there's bound to be a fair share of technical difficulties ranging from the downright annoying (yeast infections) to the long-lasting (loss of hormones due to menopause):

- **Amenorrhea:** Absence of menstrual period

- **Cervicitis:** Inflammation of the cervix

- **Dysmenorrhea:** Painful menstrual periods

- **Dyspareunia:** Painful or difficult intercourse

- **Endometritis:** Inflammation of endometrium

- **Gynatresia (atresia):** Absence of normal body opening (an *occlusion*); gynatresia usually refers to part of female genital tract, the vagina

- **HRT (hormone replacement therapy):** Replacement of hormones to treat menopausal symptoms (also called *ERT: estrogen replacement therapy*)

- **Hydrosalpinx:** Water in fallopian tube

- **Mastitis:** Inflammation of the breast occurring during breastfeeding, usually bacterial in nature

Baby steps: OB abbreviations

Things happen fast in the birthing room, so OB physicians and their employees like to use abbreviations to keep the chatting to a minimum. Some abbreviations associated with obstetrics and neonatology are as follows:

AB: Abortion

CPD: Cephalopelvic disproportion; fetal head is too large to pass through the mother's pelvis

CS or C-section: Cesarean section

DOB: Date of birth

EDC: Expected date of confinement or delivery (due date)

FHS: Fetal heart sounds

LMP: Last menstrual period; date that last menstrual period began

NB: Newborn

OB: Obstetrics

RDS: Respiratory distress syndrome

SFH: Symphysis-fundus height, measurement taken from *symphysis pubis* (pubic bone) to *fundus* (highest level) of uterus; provides a growth record of the uterine fundus as a pregnancy progresses

- ✔ **Menometrorrhagia:** Excessive menstrual flow both during and between menstrual periods

- ✔ **Menorrhagia:** Heavy menstrual period

- ✔ **Oophoritis:** Inflammation of ovary

- ✔ **PMD (premenstrual dysphoric syndrome):** Used to describe severe premenstrual syndrome, which results in a week or two of hormonally triggered clinical depression every month

- ✔ **PMS (premenstrual syndrome):** Cyclic disorder involving physical and emotional symptoms in the premenstrual phase (just before menses phase); symptoms include fatigue, bloating, tension, and irritability

- ✔ **Vaginitis:** Inflammation of the vagina

Some conditions of the female reproductive system are specifically related to pregnancy and childbirth:

- ✔ **Abruptio placentae:** Premature separation of placenta from the uterine wall causing bleeding and a rigid, painful abdomen and requiring emergency cesarean section

- ✔ **Dystocia:** Difficult labor

- ✔ **Eclampsia:** Severe complication of pregnancy involving convulsions and/or coma in a pregnant female

- ✔ **Ectopic pregnancy:** Pregnancy occurring outside the uterus (*tubal pregnancy*) requiring emergency surgery

- ✔ **Intrauterine fetal death:** Fetal death occurring before expected date of birth

- ✔ **Missed abortion:** A fetal demise has occurred but miscarriage by expulsion has not taken place

- ✔ **Placenta previa:** Placenta develops in the lower uterine wall and may cover the cervix, blocking the birth canal and requiring a C-section; can be diagnosed by ultrasound

- ✔ **Preeclampsia:** Condition during pregnancy or shortly after delivery with high blood pressure, *edema* (swelling), and protein in the urine

- ✔ **Salpingocyesis:** Pregnancy occurring in fallopian tube or ectopic pregnancy

- ✔ **Spontaneous abortion:** A miscarriage, usually occurring before 12 weeks of gestation

- ✔ **Stillbirth:** Fetal death occurring just prior to time of delivery

Finding the Culprit: Female Reproductive Diseases and Pathology

It's important to note that the following conditions not only influence the work of the body, but also the overall mental health of the women they affect. As with the male reproductive system, a woman's mental and sexual health are intricately interwoven with physical health. For many women, issues involving reproductive health often have long-lasting effects on feminine and sexual identity. This is especially true if it affects a woman's ability to conceive or involves loss of reproductive organs, so these diseases and pathological conditions should be addressed with the utmost care and sensitivity.

- **Adenomyosis** refers to endometrium growth in the myometrium of the uterus.

- **Breast carcinoma** is a malignant tumor of the breast. Tumors may spread to skin, chest wall, and lymph nodes located in axilla; they may metastasize (spread) to other parts of the body including bones, lungs, liver, brain, and even ovaries. Breast carcinoma can be treated in a variety of ways, including *lumpectomy* (removal of cancerous lump only), removal of breast tissue but preserving skin and nipple for future reconstruction (*subcutaneous mastectomy*), removal of the entire breast (a simple or total mastectomy), or removal of breast, lymph nodes, and adjacent chest wall muscle in a single procedure (radical mastectomy).

- **Carcinoma of cervix** means malignant tumor of the cervix. *Papanicolaou (Pap) smear* detects early *cervical neoplasia* by microscopic examination of cells scraped from *cervical epithelium*.

- **Endometrial carcinoma** refers to malignant tumor of the uterus.

- **Endometriosis** involves endometrial tissue in an abnormal location, such as the ovaries or intestine, associated with dysmenorrhea, pelvic pain, and infertility.

- **Fibrocystic disease** is a disease of the breast. It is a benign condition involving one or more tumors of the breast.

- **Fibroid (leiomyoma)** is a benign tumor in the uterus composed of fibrous tissue and muscle, may cause pelvic pain or menorrhagia.

- **Ovarian cyst** is collections of fluid within a sac or cyst in the ovary.

- **Ovarian carcinoma** means malignant tumor of the ovary (*adenocarcinoma*). It may be cystic or solid.

- **PID (pelvic inflammatory disease)** refers to inflammation of female pelvic organs.

- **Prolapsed uterus** involves displacement of uterus down into the vagina.

- **Stein-Leventhal syndrome (polycystic ovary syndrome)** refers to adrenal gland malfunction resulting in facial hair (*hirsutism*), weight gain, and infrequent, abnormal, or absent menstrual periods.

- **TSS (toxic shock syndrome)** is a severe illness caused by bacterial infection, most often seen in menstruating women using tampons. Staphylococcus aureus is the bacterial culprit.

- **Vesicovaginal fistula** is when there is an opening between vagina and urinary bladder.

Testing, Testing: Female Reproductive Radiology and Diagnostic Tests

Thank goodness for modern medicine. It certainly helps ease the mind of many a woman by providing answers to the most pressing female reproductive questions. Most women will be familiar with some of these yearly (or more often for some) tests that, although causing a bit of discomfort at the time, give great comfort in the long run by offering diagnoses for many serious conditions.

- **Hysterosalpingogram:** X-ray taken of the uterus and fallopian tubes after a dye is introduced in the uterus to see if it can move freely through the fallopian tubes and out to the ovaries; used to diagnose blockages in tubes that might lead to infertility

- **Papanicolaou (Pap) smear:** Sample of cells of cervix are harvested and examined under microscopic analysis; the presence of cervical or vaginal carcinoma can be detected

- **Pregnancy test:** Detects the presence of HCG in the urine or blood to diagnose pregnancy

- **Mammogram:** X-ray film of the breast

- **Sonohysterography:** Recording uterus by sound waves (ultrasound)

Paging Dr. Terminology: Female Reproductive Surgeries and Procedures

Now that you're in tune with the working parts and possible issues involved with the female reproductive system, it's time to find out more about the things your physician can do to fix the feminine plumbing, so to speak. Obviously, many of these surgeries and procedures involve a woman's ability to conceive, whether it be putting an end to that ability through a hysterectomy or helping improve a woman's chances to get pregnant. First, let's talk about some general procedures.

- ✔ **Abortion** is the termination of a pregnancy before the embryo or the fetus is able to exist on its own. A spontaneous abortion may occur in a pregnancy up to and including 12 weeks, and is also known as a *miscarriage*. A therapeutic or induced abortion is a deliberate termination of pregnancy and is most commonly performed during the first trimester between 8 and 12 weeks.

- ✔ **Cervical conization** is a cone-shaped biopsy of tissue from the mouth of cervix for diagnostic purposes. This procedure often follows an abnormal Pap smear.

- ✔ **Cryosurgery:** This refers to the use of cold or freezing temperature to destroy tissue, usually produced by a probe containing liquid nitrogen.

- ✔ **D & C** means dilatation and curettage. First, the *dilatation* (widening of the cervical opening) is accomplished. *Curettage* (scraping) is accomplished next by using a curette or metal loop to remove samples of the lining of the uterus for diagnostic purposes. Also performed to remove products of conception after an incomplete miscarriage or to reduce uterine bleeding.

- ✔ **Hysteroscopy** is visual examination of the uterus performed with a *hysteroscope*.

Many women opt for a permanent form of sterilization once they make the decision to not have more (or any) children. The procedures are very common, and each has its own set of pros and cons. Women are typically encouraged to choose the sterilization method best for their individual lifestyles and physical makeup. A very common sterilization method is *tubal ligation*, a procedure that involves cutting or interrupting and *ligating* (tying off) fallopian tubes to prevent passage of ovum. This procedure can be done laparoscopically or through an abdominal incision:

- ✔ **Laparoscopic method:** Laparoscope is inserted through the abdominal wall, and tubes can be sealed off with high-frequency spark (*cauterization*) or burning.

- ✔ **Tubal banding:** A band is wrapped around a section of each tube and tissue becomes *necrotic* (dies), providing a break between the two portions of tube.

- ✔ **Tubal clipping:** *Filshie clip* is used to clip off tubes, similar to banding method.

Having fun with hormones: Beginning to end and birth control in between

Menstruation and pregnancy not only depend on the hormones produced in the ovaries, but also on hormones secreted from the pituitary gland. *Follicle-stimulating hormones (FSH)* and *luteinizing hormones (LH)* help stimulate the development of the ovum and ovulation. After ovulation, LH influences the maintenance of the corpus luteum and its production of estrogen and progesterone.

During pregnancy the higher levels of estrogen and progesterone affect the pituitary gland itself, by shedding off its production of FSH and LH. When a woman is pregnant then, new ova do not mature, and ovulation cannot occur. This interaction, when hormones act to shut off the production of another group of hormones, is called *negative feedback*. This is the principle behind the action of birth control pills on the body. The *birth control pill* contains varying amounts of estrogen and progesterone, causing the hormone levels to rise in the blood. Negative feedback occurs, and the pituitary does not release FSH and LH. Ovulation cannot occur without these, and a woman cannot become pregnant.

Other female contraceptive measures include the IUD (intrauterine device) and the diaphragm. The *IUD* is a small coil placed inside the uterus by a physician. Its presence in the uterus (foreign body) irritates the uterine lining to prevent implantation of a fertilized ovum. A *diaphragm* is a rubber cup-shaped device inserted over the outside of the cervix before intercourse to prevent sperm from entering the cervix and moving into the uterus to the fallopian tubes.

The finale of this ongoing cycle occurs when the secretion of estrogen from the ovaries lessens, fewer eggs are produced, and menopause begins. *Menopause* is the gradual ending of the menstrual cycle and the natural process resulting from normal aging of the ovaries. Other names for menopause are "change of life" and "climacteric." Premature menopause can occur before age 35, whereas delayed menopause can occur after age 55. Artificial menopause occurs if the ovaries are removed surgically or made nonfunctional by radiation therapy. Menopause is considered complete when menstrual periods have been absent for at least 12 months.

Laparoscopic tubal ligations were done in the 1970s, and the first *laparoscopic cholecystectomy* was performed in 1989.

Many surgical procedures for the female reproductive system require the repair or removal of some parts of the system. In the most serious cases (often involving cancer), the entire uterus and surrounding cervix are completely removed. Keep in mind that breasts are considered part of this system as well, so in the following list you'll see terms referring to the surgical removal or repair of these body parts as well.

✔ **Abdominal hysterectomy:** Surgical removal of the uterus through the abdomen

✔ **Bilateral salpingo-oophorectomy:** Surgical removal of both tubes and both ovaries

- ✔ **Colpopexy:** Surgical fixation of the vagina to surrounding structures

- ✔ **Combination special (total hysterectomy and bilateral salpingo-oophorectomy):** Removal of uterus, cervix, both tubes, and ovaries; commonly referred to as *TAH-BSO (Total Abdominal Hysterectomy with Bilateral Salpingo-Oophorectomy)*

- ✔ **Hymenectomy:** Surgical removal of the hymen

- ✔ **Hysteropexy:** Surgical fixation of a misplaced or abnormally mobile uterus

- ✔ **Laparoscopic hysterectomy:** Surgical removal of the uterus using a laparoscope

- ✔ **Lumpectomy:** Removal of cancerous lump only in the breast; subcutaneous mastectomy is removal of breast tissue that preserves skin and nipple for future reconstruction; simple or total mastectomy may involve removal of the entire breast; in a radical mastectomy, the breast is removed, along with the lymph nodes and adjacent chest wall muscle in a single procedure

- ✔ **Mastectomy:** Surgical removal of a breast

- ✔ **Oophorectomy:** Surgical removal of an ovary

- ✔ **Salpingectomy:** Surgical removal of a fallopian tube

- ✔ **Salpingo-oophorectomy (or oophoro-salpingectomy):** Removal of fallopian tube and ovary

- ✔ **Subtotal hysterectomy:** Surgical removal of uterus only (cervix left behind)

- ✔ **Total hysterectomy:** Surgical removal of uterus and cervix

- ✔ **Vaginal hysterectomy:** Uterus and cervix are surgically removed via vagina

- ✔ **Vaginoplasty:** Surgical repair of the vagina

- ✔ **Vulvectomy:** Surgical removal of the vulva

Of course, because creating life and giving birth are two huge jobs of this system, you would be remiss to miss these obstetrical terms:

- ✔ **Amniotomy**: Incision into the amnion to induce labor. It's also referred to as *artificial rupture of membranes.*

- ✔ **Cesarean section:** This is surgical removal of the fetus through the abdominal and uterine walls. A *C-section* may be performed for a *breech* presentation (baby's head is not in downward position), multiple births, *placenta previa (*placenta develops in the lower uterine wall and may cover the cervix, blocking the birth canal*), abruptio placentae* (premature separation of placenta from uterine wall), *cephalopelvic disproportion* (when a baby's head or body is too large to fit through the mother's pelvis), failure to progress in labor, or any sign that the fetus is in distress.

- **Episiotomy:** Refers to incision of vulva or perineum. This is done during delivery to prevent tearing of the perineum.

- **Amniocentesis:** This involves surgical puncture to aspirate amniotic fluid via insertion of needle through the abdominal and uterine walls using ultrasound guidance. Fluid is used for the assessment of fetal health and maturity. This procedure is used to aid in diagnosis of fetal abnormalities. It is performed early in pregnancy at 16 weeks to determine fetal abnormalities such as *Down syndrome*, *spina bifida*, or to determine the sex of the fetus. It is done late in the pregnancy to determine lung maturity of the fetus.

- **Pelvimetry:** The measurement of the mother's pelvic to determine ability of fetus to pass through.

- **Obstetrical ultrasound:** Ultrasound of the abdomen and pelvis determine fetal development, growth rate, and estimate fetal age, weight, and maturity.

- **Salpingectomy:** Removal of a fallopian tube in order to remove an ectopic pregnancy.

Terminology RX: Female Reproductive Pharmacology

And now for a brief word about our friends, the drugs. Many women hoping to have children who are experiencing difficulties are very thankful to have drugs to treat fertility, such as *clomiphene citrate*. These little wonders work by stimulating the pituitary gland to release LH and FSH, thus increasing the body's ability to conceive. Though these drugs are not panaceas, they have helped countless women reach their goals of becoming mothers. On the other end of the conception spectrum, some babies want to make their appearance too early. In these cases, uterine relaxants are used to stop premature labor in pregnancy.

Analgesics are painkillers used to treat menstrual cramps and painful periods. Then there are the "antis." *Antifungal drugs* are used to treat vaginal yeast infections, whereas *anti-inflammatories* and *antibiotics* are used to treat some sexually transmitted diseases. (For more information about STDs that affect both woman and men, see Chapter 22.)

Part VI
The Part of Tens

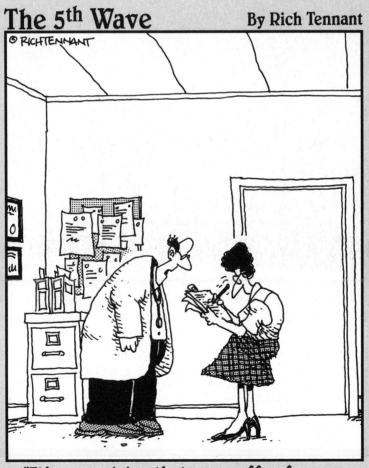

The 5th Wave   By Rich Tennant

"It's my opinion that you suffer from a hyperactive disorder. And when you're done writing that down, I'd like my chart back."

In this part . . .

This is the quick and dirty section. Get your mind out of the gutter! We just mean that this is a section full of quick, easy-to-learn information that will sharpen your terminology-addled brain and impress people at dinner parties. In Chapter 24, you get a quick list of our favorite terminology resources, from books to Web sites. Chapter 25 shows you some cool mnemonic devices, while Chapter 26 gives you ideas for fun word-building activities for those days when flashcards just won't do.

Chapter 24

Ten Essential Medical Terminology References

In This Chapter

▶ Access the most widely used terminology references

▶ Find the type of reference that works best for your lifestyle

*O*h, you know you want more. Medical terminology references, that is. What did you think we meant? Whether you are drawn to the stacks at your local library or prefer the click of the computer keyboard, here are ten terminology references that you can't live without.

Medterms.com

A subset site of MedicineNet.com, this medical reference includes over 16,000 terms. Via a simple search engine, the site can look for words of similar spelling and incorrect spelling — which is a boon for those of us who never won a spelling bee. The site also offers a word of the day and earns its street cred by the fact that its doctors authored the latest edition of the *Webster's New World Medical Dictionary*.

Medilexicon.com

This Web site is a good all-arounder, featuring a fully searchable list of medical abbreviations and a medical dictionary. It's a searchapalooza, offering search functions for drugs, medical instruments, and ICD-9 codes (codes used for medical charting and billing).

Merriam-Webster's Medical Desk Dictionary

This desk reference comes to you courtesy of big daddy Merriam-Webster. You've heard of Merriam-Webster, right? These darlings of diction have written their fair share of word references, so you're certainly in good hands.

webMD.com

You can always count on webMD.com to provide the latest cutting-edge medical news and information. And, yes, you can also drive yourself insane using the Symptom Checker to pinpoint what ails you. (Once you start, you'll do it every time you feel a sniffle coming on.) In addition to the latest news, you can search for doctors, hospitals, drugs, and practically every medical topic known to man. Connect to blogs, message boards, expert forums, and even health quizzes, games, and slideshows.

Dorland's Illustrated Medical Dictionary

If you consider yourself a visual learner, consider Dorland's your new best friend. Not only does this dictionary have all of the terms you need to know, it offers full illustrations to help get the point across. And, it's available both online at `www.dorlands.com` and in hardcopy format.

Mosby's Medical Dictionary

This monster is well over 2,000 pages chocked full of medical terminology know-how. It includes a thumb-indexed dictionary and tons of illustrations to help you visualize the terms as actual body parts. Not exactly something you want to carry around in your book bag, but definitely handy to keep on your bookshelf. Plus, it makes a great doorstop or paperweight. Mosby's is famous for the number of colored pictures, which tends to be helpful for the novice medical terminology student.

Stedman's Medical Dictionary and Flashcards for Health Professionals and Nursing Illustrated, 5th Edition

This particular book is the major reference from this publisher, but the company also offers tons of smaller, more precise references if you want to narrow down your stack of books a bit. From illustrated flashcards and skill-building tools to guides to idioms, terms, and phrases, *Stedman's* is a one-stop shop for all things terminology. And, of course, they offer tons of online resources at www.stedmans.com as well if you want to travel light.

Taber's Cyclopedic Medical Dictionary

Taber's Web site at www.tabers.com says that it is the "world's best-selling health-sciences dictionary," offering over 56,000 terms. Like many of its competitors, *Taber's* offers not only the print version of its dictionary, but also a Web component and terms sent directly to your PDA or wireless handheld device. *Taber's* other vital stats include: 700 full-color images, 2500 audio pronunciations, customized bookmarking, "sounds like" search, and topic cross-linking. So, if you're checking out one particular part of a system, *Taber's* will point you in the direction of related information. That's a nice little bit of handholding.

Medicalmnemonics.com

This is a cool and fun Web site. If you need a little boost to help you remember words and terms, chances are you already use mnemonic devices. You know, like "I before E, except after C, or when sounding like A as in neighbor and weigh."

Mnemonics are often simple little phrases to help you recall what it is you're trying to learn and put on paper, into speech, or fill in on a standardized test. This is a whole Web site dedicated to the concept. Working much like a wiki, *you* can add your own devices to the database and help others. You can search the database (of course) or browse by systems and charts. You can even customize to fit your needs or set the site up to download to your phone or PDA. The coolest part is: It's totally free and not-for-profit. So thank your fellow medheads for sharing the love, and remember to share some yourself by adding your own useful mnemonics.

Medical Terminology Systems Quick Study Guide

The good folks at Bar Charts, Inc. figured, eh, why bother with all of the pages and binding that ties down a traditional book! When you really want to know something, you want it to magically appear right before your eyes. Voilá! Enter the *Quick Study Guide*, also known as the giant laminated poster. You've probably seen similar charts in the doctor's office showcasing your insides. This one is super handy and hits the terminology highlights. You can find all sorts of similar guides at www.barcharts.com for things like common abbreviations, individual systems terms (with illustrations), and even guides just for nurses. Who needs wallpaper when you can hang these babies up?

Chapter 25

Ten or So Useful
Mnemonic Devices

▶ Using simple phrasing devices to remember medical terms.

▶ Discovering quick ways to recall simple system functions.

A *mnemonic device* is any kind of simple way to remember something, such as lists of terms, functions, or definitions. They are usually kind of silly, which makes them stand out in your mind. In this chapter we've compiled eleven great useful devices from one of our favorite Web sites, www. medicalmnemonics.com (see Chapter 24 for more info on this cool site).

Cranial Nerves

Don't strain your cranium to recall those cranial nerves. Just remember: "On Old Olympus Towering Top, A Finn And German Viewed Some Hops" to recall these nerves: olfactory, optic, oculomotor, trochlear, trigeminal, abducens, facial, auditory-vestibular, glossopharyngeal, vagus, spinal accessory, and hypoglossal.

Lung Lobe Numbers

To remember the location of the different sides of the lungs, think *tri* and *bi*. The tri-lobed lung lives on the right side, along with the tricuspid heart valve. The bicuspid and bi-lobed lung live on the left side of your body.

The Size of a Thyroid

Ever play that game where you look at the clouds and try to figure out what they look like? Well, you can do the same with the thyroid, which looks a little bit like a bra. To remember the size of the thyroid, just remember that breasts are bigger in women than men, so the thyroid is bigger in women. Even more, pregnant women have the largest breasts, and they also have the largest thyroids.

Scalp Layers

The layers of your scalp actually spell SCALP. Remember this easy formula:

Skin

Connective tissue

Aponeurosis

Loose Connective Tissue

Pericranium

SCALP!

Muscles of the Rotator Cuff

Rotator cuff injuries can be debilitating, especially for an athlete. You can remember the muscles of the rotator cuff by remembering SITS. These muscles are (clockwise from top): Supraspinatus, Infraspinatus, Teres minor, and Subscapularis.

Note: If a baseball pitcher injures these muscles, he SITS out for the rest of the game.

Radial Nerve

The muscles supplied by the radial nerve are the BEST! Remember:

> **B**rachioradialis
>
> **E**xtensors
>
> **S**upinator
>
> **T**riceps

BEST!

Face Nerves

You can recall what the major face muscles do by matching the action to the name. Think *M* and *Facial*. The *mandibular* nerve is in charge of *mastication*. The *facial* nerve is in charge of *facial expression*.

Perineal versus Peroneal

Can't keep these two words straight? Just remember that perIN eal is *in between* the legs. PerONeal is *on* the legs.

Sperm Path through Male Reproductive Tract

Poor Steve. He gets a tough break here, but he's the best candidate for remembering the path sperm takes to exit the male body. Meet Steve:

> **S**eminiferous Tubules
>
> **E**pididymis
>
> **V**as deferens
>
> **E**jaculatory duct

Carpal Bone Locations

Who knew the carpal bones could be so racy? When you're trying to think of these bones, consider that *Some Lovers Try Positions That They Can't Handle*:

Scaphoid

Lunate

Triquetrum

Pisiform

Trapezium

Trapezoid

Capitate

Hamate

Cranial Bones

Since cranial bones help make up your skull, keep skulls in mind to recall the bones and think "Old Pygmies From Thailand Eat Skulls":

Occipital

Parietal

Frontal

Temporal

Ethmoid

Sphenoid

Chapter 26

Ten Fun Word-Building Activities

▶ Creating some fun alternatives to memorization

▶ Finding the activity that best helps you remember important terms

*L*et's face it: Memorizing lists of medical terms is probably not the most fun activity you'll ever do. Are there ways to spice it up? As it turns out, there are. And here is where we share them with you.

Word Grouping

One of these things is quite like the other. Okay, that's not how the song goes, but it serves your purposes if you remember terms best by grouping them into similar categories. Many times, it helps you remember if you think about terms in relation to similar terms. You can group words and terms by

✔ System

✔ Function

✔ Sound

✔ Prefixes or Suffixes

✔ Common roots

✔ Word type (such body part, condition, disease, procedure, or pharmacology)

The possibilities are endless, so spend some time thinking about what works best for you.

Using Medical Word Parts You Already Know to Build Words

Have a great sense of recall? Latch your brain onto some word parts that make natural sense to you and then start building words. Some prefixes, for example, are pretty self-explanatory. Cardio is for heart. Gyne/o is for all things femininely reproductive. So use what comes naturally to learn the related words.

Here's one method:

1. Start by listing the word parts you already know through everyday use, even what you know from television programs. Just make sure they are correct!

2. Create a worksheet for each word part you know. You can do this in a notebook, in a word-processing program, or — even more efficiently — in a spreadsheet format.

3. Build some words! Just go freeform at this point and add all the related words you know.

4. Once you've got the lists started, you can start researching more words derived from that root, prefix, or suffix. By the time you're ready to study, you'll have a mega database of words.

Matching the Word Part to the Definition

A similar activity involves matching the word part, whether it be prefix, suffix, or root, to its definition. This is probably the most standard form of memorization, but it works. If you can learn those individual word parts, you can create darn near any medical term. Here is one low-tech, useful way to do this:

Create two sets of flashcards — one with the word part and one with the corresponding definition. Then work to match them up. How do you know if you're right? Cut each card in half in a distinctive way so that it will fit together with its partner. If it fits, you've done it!

Crosswords

Are you one of those people who spend Sunday mornings knee-deep in newspapers, working the jumble or crossword? Consider yourself a master word builder? Well, this fun and mentally challenging activity isn't just a great way to kill a few hours, it's a terrific way to remember words and their definitions. You can either create your own crossword or look to other resources to find them. To create your own, check out DIY sites like the following:

✔ www.crosswordpuzzlegames.com

✔ www.armoredpenguin.com/crossword/

✔ www.edhelper.com/crossword.htm

You can also purchase DIY crossword software from sites like http:// puzzlemaker.discoveryeducation.com.

If you're not up to creating your own crosswords, here are a couple online resources:

✔ www.studystack.com

✔ www.medword.com

Also check out medical institution Web sites. Many programs offer word-building games and puzzles to both students and visitors.

Flashcards

There are tons of great flashcard products on the market (see Chapter 25 for some of the most common), or you can go old school and make your own. All you need is cheapo packet of index cards and a marker and you're in business. You can do them by definition, system, function, or word part.

Name That System

If you can name a function, you can name a system. Set up this activity with some friends and margaritas, and you have a full night of fun. This activity can be done in a variety of ways, from basic Q&A to a *Jeopardy*-like format. You can incorporate some quick and easy flashcards with this as well. A similar activity is to rattle off a bunch of terms and name the system associated with them, or do the exact opposite.

Medical Hangman

You remember killing time playing hangman, don't you? This is exactly the same activity, but with medical terms. And maybe the little man drawing isn't hanging, but instead is lying on the operating table. Here are a few sites that provide medical hangman games:

- ✔ www.quia.com
- ✔ www.studystack.com
- ✔ www.cssolutions.biz

Word Search

Create a word search out of terms you need to know. There are several computer programs that offer word search creation tools, and many are free online. Set up a search using any terms you need to know. This activity works best if you use words that are unfamiliar or hard to remember. Where's the challenge in finding words you know well? Stretch yourself and see what happens. Try these sites:

- ✔ www.edhelper.com
- ✔ www.armoredpenguin.com/wordsearch/
- ✔ http://teachers.teach-nology.com/web_tools/word_search/

You can also try some Web sites with already-created medical word searches:

- ✔ www.mwsearch.com
- ✔ www.world-english.org/wordsearchmedical.htm
- ✔ www.medword.com
- ✔ www.medtrng.com/quia.htm

Combining Forms

Our good buddies, the combining forms (root words), are back. You can create customized lists of combining forms along with their definitions, mix and match, or get a roommate or significant other to quiz you (or simply quiz yourself) on meanings.

Jumble

A completely maddening, time-consuming, and highly useful word-building activity is the *word jumble*. This is exactly what it sounds like. Words are jumbled, letters are mixed up, and it's your duty to create a real word from the mess. For example, can you make sense out of *etrvidluiucsiti*? It's good old *diverticulitis* in disguise! Word jumbles are incredibly useful if you have issues with spelling and work beautifully with very long words. Jumble.com and wordjumble.com are two of the most popular sites.

Appendix

Prefixes and Suffixes

• •

In This Chapter

▶ Kicking things off with prefixes

▶ Closing things out with suffixes

• •

*N*eed a quick fix? Here is a grand list of the major prefixes and suffixes we cover in the book, all alphabetized and ready to be studied. Many of these can be applied to more than one body system.

Quickly, before you dive into the prefixes and suffixes you've come to know and love, think about what each word part does and why it does it. Prefixes and suffixes are modifiers or adjectives that alter the meaning of the root word, in the same ways as regular English terms.

The beginning, the alpha, the jumping-off point is the prefix. The prefix tells you something about what you are going to find inside the word itself. A prefix appears at the beginning of a word and tells the how, why, where, when, how much, how many, position, direction, time, or status.

You might recognize many of the prefixes associated with medical terminology, because they have similar meanings in regular, everyday vernacular. For example, the most basic prefix of *a-* means without, or not, in medical terminology, just as it does in any other word. If something is *atypical*, for example, it is not typical. *Hemi-* means half, as in *hemisphere*. The moral of this story is that prefixes aren't just window dressing. They have a unique and specific goal, which is to tell you more about the circumstances surrounding the word's meaning.

Prefixes

A-/ or an-/	Without or lack of
Bi- or bin-	Two
Brady	Slow
Dys-	Difficult, painful, uncomfortable
Endo-	Within
Epi-	On, over, upon
Eu-	Normal
Ex-, exo-	Outside, outward
Hemi-	Half
Hydro-	Water
Hyper -	Excessive, above normal
Hypo-	Below normal
Inter-	Between
Intra-	Within
Nulli-	None
Pan-	All
Para-	Abnormal
Para-	Beside, beyond, around
per	Through
Peri-	Around
Polio-	Gray
Poly	Many, much
Primi-	First
Quadri-	Four
Re-	Back
Retro -	Backward, back
Secundi-	Second
Sub-	Below, under
Tachy-	Fast
Trans-	Through or across
Trans-	Through, across, beyond

Suffixes

Next we have the omega, the last call of the word scene — the suffix. The suffix, always at the end of a word, usually indicates a procedure, a condition, or a disease. Whereas the prefix gives us a clue into what to expect in a word's meaning, the suffix pulls no punches and tells us what is happening with a specific body part or system. And usually it either entails what is wrong medically or indicates the procedure used to diagnose or fix it.

Suffixes operate in the medical world much as they do in the land of standard English. Like prefixes, many of these have similar meanings in plain old, everyday English that you hear on the street. For example, the suffix *-meter* simply indicates an instrument used to measure something, just as it does in English (like *odometer*). *Geography*, a term feared by many fifth graders the world over, ends with *-graphy* and means, more or less, "picturing lands."

-algia	Pain
-apheresis	Removal
-ar, -ary	Pertaining to
-ase	Enzyme
-blast	Immature
-capnia	Carbon dioxide
-centesis	Surgical puncture with needle to aspirate fluid
-chalasis	Relaxation
-continence	To stop
-cusis	Hearing
-cyesis	Pregnancy
-cytosis	Condition of cells
-desis	Surgical fixation
-drome	Run, running
-ectasis	Stretching or expansion
-ectomy	Surgical removal or excision
-emia	A blood condition
-flux	Flow
-gen	Producing
-genesis	Production
-globin	Protein
-globulin	Protein
-gram	Picture or finished record
-graph	Instrument used to record

-graphy	Process of recording
-iasis	Abnormal condition
-ician	One who
-ism	State of or condition
-itis	Inflammation
-lithiasis	Calculus or stone
-lysis	Loosening, separating
-lytic	Destruction or breakdown
-malacia	Softening
-megaly	Enlargement
-metrist	Specialist in the measurement of
-metry	Process of measuring
-ology	Study of
-oma	Tumor or mass
-opia	Vision (condition)
-opsy	View of, viewing
-optosis	Sagging
-orrhaphy	Surgical fixation or suturing
-orrhea	Flow, excessive discharge
-ory	Pertaining to
-oscopy	Visual examination of internal cavity using a scope
-ostomy	Creation of an artificial opening
-otomy	Process of cutting into
-oxia	Oxygen
-para	To bear, live birth
-paresis	Slight paralysis
-pathy	Disease
-pepsia	Digestion
-pexy	Surgical fixation
-phagia	Eating or swallowing
-phonia	Sound
-phoresis	Carrying/transmission
-plasty	Surgical repair or reconstruction
-plegia	Paralysis
-pnea	Breathing
-poiesis	Formation
-prandial	Meal
-ptosis	Drooping, sagging, prolapse
-rrhagia	Burst forth, excessive flow

-rrhaphy	Suture repair
-rrhea	Discharge or flow
-salpinx	Fallopian tube
-schisis	Cleft or splitting
-scope	Instrument used to visually examine
-scopy	Visual examination
-stasis	Stop or control
-stenosis	Narrowing or constricting
-thenia	Lack of strength
-thorax	Chest
-tocia	Labor
-tresia	Opening
-tripsy	Surgical crushing
-tropia	To turn
-uria	Urination, urine
-us	Condition

Index

• **P** •

BUSINESS, CAREERS & PERSONAL FINANCE

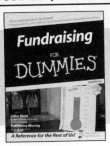

Fundraising FOR DUMMIES
0-7645-9847-3

Investing FOR DUMMIES
0-7645-2431-3

Also available:

- Business Plans Kit For Dummies
  0-7645-9794-9
- Economics For Dummies
  0-7645-5726-2
- Grant Writing For Dummies
  0-7645-8416-2
- Home Buying For Dummies
  0-7645-5331-3
- Managing For Dummies
  0-7645-1771-6
- Marketing For Dummies
  0-7645-5600-2

- Personal Finance For Dummies
  0-7645-2590-5*
- Resumes For Dummies
  0-7645-5471-9
- Selling For Dummies
  0-7645-5363-1
- Six Sigma For Dummies
  0-7645-6798-5
- Small Business Kit For Dummies
  0-7645-5984-2
- Starting an eBay Business For Dummies
  0-7645-6924-4
- Your Dream Career For Dummies
  0-7645-9795-7

HOME & BUSINESS COMPUTER BASICS

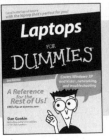

Laptops FOR DUMMIES
0-470-05432-8

Windows Vista FOR DUMMIES
0-471-75421-8

Also available:

- Cleaning Windows Vista For Dummies
  0-471-78293-9
- Excel 2007 For Dummies
  0-470-03737-7
- Mac OS X Tiger For Dummies
  0-7645-7675-5
- MacBook For Dummies
  0-470-04859-X
- Macs For Dummies
  0-470-04849-2
- Office 2007 For Dummies
  0-470-00923-3

- Outlook 2007 For Dummies
  0-470-03830-6
- PCs For Dummies
  0-7645-8958-X
- Salesforce.com For Dummies
  0-470-04893-X
- Upgrading & Fixing Laptops For Dummies
  0-7645-8959-8
- Word 2007 For Dummies
  0-470-03658-3
- Quicken 2007 For Dummies
  0-470-04600-7

FOOD, HOME, GARDEN, HOBBIES, MUSIC & PETS

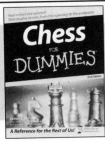

Chess FOR DUMMIES
0-7645-8404-9

Guitar FOR DUMMIES
0-7645-9904-6

Also available:

- Candy Making For Dummies
  0-7645-9734-5
- Card Games For Dummies
  0-7645-9910-0
- Crocheting For Dummies
  0-7645-4151-X
- Dog Training For Dummies
  0-7645-8418-9
- Healthy Carb Cookbook For Dummies
  0-7645-8476-6
- Home Maintenance For Dummies
  0-7645-5215-5

- Horses For Dummies
  0-7645-9797-3
- Jewelry Making & Beading For Dummies
  0-7645-2571-9
- Orchids For Dummies
  0-7645-6759-4
- Puppies For Dummies
  0-7645-5255-4
- Rock Guitar For Dummies
  0-7645-5356-9
- Sewing For Dummies
  0-7645-6847-7
- Singing For Dummies
  0-7645-2475-5

INTERNET & DIGITAL MEDIA

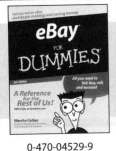

eBay FOR DUMMIES
0-470-04529-9

iPod & iTunes FOR DUMMIES
0-470-04894-8

Also available:

- Blogging For Dummies
  0-471-77084-1
- Digital Photography For Dummies
  0-7645-9802-3
- Digital Photography All-in-One Desk Reference For Dummies
  0-470-03743-1
- Digital SLR Cameras and Photography For Dummies
  0-7645-9803-1
- eBay Business All-in-One Desk Reference For Dummies
  0-7645-8438-3
- HDTV For Dummies
  0-470-09673-X

- Home Entertainment PCs For Dummie
  0-470-05523-5
- MySpace For Dummies
  0-470-09529-6
- Search Engine Optimization For Dummies
  0-471-97998-8
- Skype For Dummies
  0-470-04891-3
- The Internet For Dummies
  0-7645-8996-2
- Wiring Your Digital Home For Dummie
  0-471-91830-X

* Separate Canadian edition also available
† Separate U.K. edition also available

Available wherever books are sold. For more information or to order direct: U.S. customers visit www.dummies.com or call 1-877-762-2974.
U.K. customers visit www.wileyeurope.com or call 0800 243407. Canadian customers visit www.wiley.ca or call 1-800-567-4797.

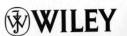 WILEY

SPORTS, FITNESS, PARENTING, RELIGION & SPIRITUALITY

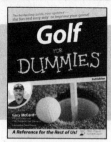

0-471-76871-5

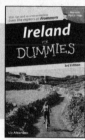

0-7645-7841-3

Also available:
- Catholicism For Dummies
  0-7645-5391-7
- Exercise Balls For Dummies
  0-7645-5623-1
- Fitness For Dummies
  0-7645-7851-0
- Football For Dummies
  0-7645-3936-1
- Judaism For Dummies
  0-7645-5299-6
- Potty Training For Dummies
  0-7645-5417-4
- Buddhism For Dummies
  0-7645-5359-3

- Pregnancy For Dummies
  0-7645-4483-7 †
- Ten Minute Tone-Ups For Dummies
  0-7645-7207-5
- NASCAR For Dummies
  0-7645-7681-X
- Religion For Dummies
  0-7645-5264-3
- Soccer For Dummies
  0-7645-5229-5
- Women in the Bible For Dummies
  0-7645-8475-8

TRAVEL

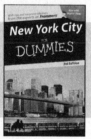

0-7645-7749-2

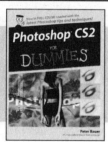

0-7645-6945-7

Also available:
- Alaska For Dummies
  0-7645-7746-8
- Cruise Vacations For Dummies
  0-7645-6941-4
- England For Dummies
  0-7645-4276-1
- Europe For Dummies
  0-7645-7529-5
- Germany For Dummies
  0-7645-7823-5
- Hawaii For Dummies
  0-7645-7402-7

- Italy For Dummies
  0-7645-7386-1
- Las Vegas For Dummies
  0-7645-7382-9
- London For Dummies
  0-7645-4277-X
- Paris For Dummies
  0-7645-7630-5
- RV Vacations For Dummies
  0-7645-4442-X
- Walt Disney World & Orlando
  For Dummies
  0-7645-9660-8

GRAPHICS, DESIGN & WEB DEVELOPMENT

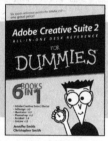

0-7645-8815-X

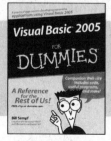

0-7645-9571-7

Also available:
- 3D Game Animation For Dummies
  0-7645-8789-7
- AutoCAD 2006 For Dummies
  0-7645-8925-3
- Building a Web Site For Dummies
  0-7645-7144-3
- Creating Web Pages For Dummies
  0-470-08030-2
- Creating Web Pages All-in-One Desk
  Reference For Dummies
  0-7645-4345-8
- Dreamweaver 8 For Dummies
  0-7645-9649-7

- InDesign CS2 For Dummies
  0-7645-9572-5
- Macromedia Flash 8 For Dummies
  0-7645-9691-8
- Photoshop CS2 and Digital
  Photography For Dummies
  0-7645-9580-6
- Photoshop Elements 4 For Dummies
  0-471-77483-9
- Syndicating Web Sites with RSS Feeds
  For Dummies
  0-7645-8848-6
- Yahoo! SiteBuilder For Dummies
  0-7645-9800-7

NETWORKING, SECURITY, PROGRAMMING & DATABASES

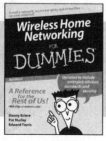

0-7645-7728-X

0-471-74940-0

Also available:
- Access 2007 For Dummies
  0-470-04612-0
- ASP.NET 2 For Dummies
  0-7645-7907-X
- C# 2005 For Dummies
  0-7645-9704-3
- Hacking For Dummies
  0-470-05235-X
- Hacking Wireless Networks
  For Dummies
  0-7645-9730-2
- Java For Dummies
  0-470-08716-1

- Microsoft SQL Server 2005 For Dummies
  0-7645-7755-7
- Networking All-in-One Desk Reference
  For Dummies
  0-7645-9939-9
- Preventing Identity Theft For Dummies
  0-7645-7336-5
- Telecom For Dummies
  0-471-77085-X
- Visual Studio 2005 All-in-One Desk
  Reference For Dummies
  0-7645-9775-2
- XML For Dummies
  0-7645-8845-1

HEALTH & SELF-HELP

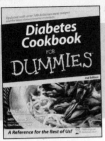

0-7645-8450-2

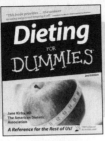

0-7645-4149-8

Also available:
- Bipolar Disorder For Dummies
  0-7645-8451-0
- Chemotherapy and Radiation For Dummies
  0-7645-7832-4
- Controlling Cholesterol For Dummies
  0-7645-5440-9
- Diabetes For Dummies
  0-7645-6820-5* †
- Divorce For Dummies
  0-7645-8417-0 †

- Fibromyalgia For Dummies
  0-7645-5441-7
- Low-Calorie Dieting For Dummies
  0-7645-9905-4
- Meditation For Dummies
  0-471-77774-9
- Osteoporosis For Dummies
  0-7645-7621-6
- Overcoming Anxiety For Dummies
  0-7645-5447-6
- Reiki For Dummies
  0-7645-9907-0
- Stress Management For Dummies
  0-7645-5144-2

EDUCATION, HISTORY, REFERENCE & TEST PREPARATION

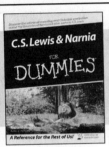

0-7645-8381-6

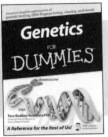

0-7645-9554-7

Also available:
- The ACT For Dummies
  0-7645-9652-7
- Algebra For Dummies
  0-7645-5325-9
- Algebra Workbook For Dummies
  0-7645-8467-7
- Astronomy For Dummies
  0-7645-8465-0
- Calculus For Dummies
  0-7645-2498-4
- Chemistry For Dummies
  0-7645-5430-1
- Forensics For Dummies
  0-7645-5580-4

- Freemasons For Dummies
  0-7645-9796-5
- French For Dummies
  0-7645-5193-0
- Geometry For Dummies
  0-7645-5324-0
- Organic Chemistry I For Dummies
  0-7645-6902-3
- The SAT I For Dummies
  0-7645-7193-1
- Spanish For Dummies
  0-7645-5194-9
- Statistics For Dummies
  0-7645-5423-9

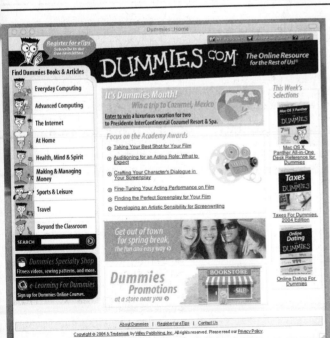

Get smart @ dummies.com®

- **Find a full list of Dummies titles**
- **Look into loads of FREE on-site articles**
- **Sign up for FREE eTips e-mailed to you weekly**
- **See what other products carry the Dummies name**
- **Shop directly from the Dummies bookstore**
- **Enter to win new prizes every month!**

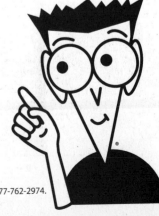

* Separate Canadian edition also available
† Separate U.K. edition also available

Available wherever books are sold. For more information or to order direct: U.S. customers visit www.dummies.com or call 1-877-762-2974.
U.K. customers visit www.wileyeurope.com or call 0800 243407. Canadian customers visit www.wiley.ca or call 1-800-567-4797.

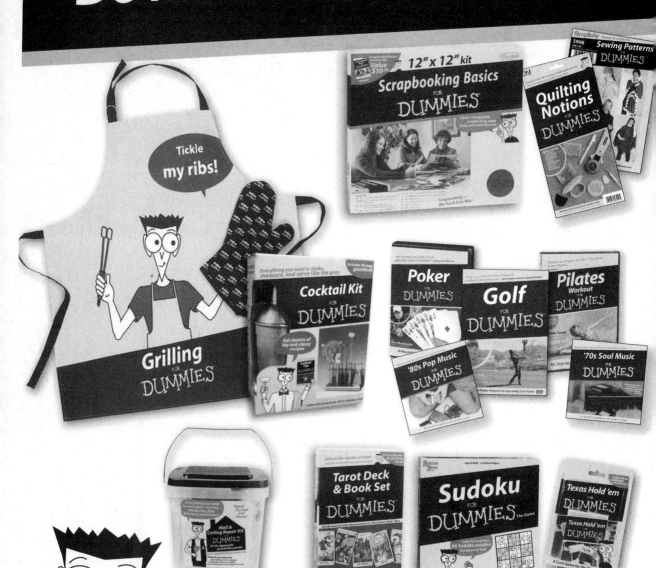
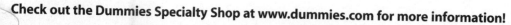
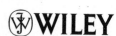